Mor

MORNING SICKNESS

A comprehensive guide to the causes and treatments

Nicky Wesson

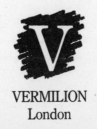

VERMILION
London

To Beverley O'Brien and Denys Fairweather
who have worked so hard in researching the
subject of pregnancy sickness, and to whom
I am indebted for their work on the history of
the subject.

1 3 5 7 9 10 8 6 4 2

Text copyright © Nicky Wesson 1997
Illustration copyright © Random House UK Ltd 1997

The right of Nicky Wesson to be identified as the author of this book has
been asserted by her in accordance with the Copyright, Designs and
Patents Act 1988.

First published in the United Kingdom in 1997 by Vermilion
an imprint of Ebury Press
Random House
20 Vauxhall Bridge Road
London SW1V 2SA

Random House Australia (Pty) Limited
20 Alfred Street, Milsons Point, Sydney,
New South Wales 2061, Australia

Random House New Zealand Limited
18 Poland Road, Glenfield,
Auckland 10, New Zealand

Random House South Africa (Pty) Ltd
Endulini, 5A Jubilee Road,
Parktown 2193, South Africa

Random House UK Limited Reg. No. 954009

A CIP catalogue record for this book is available from the British Library

ISBN: 0 09 181538 X

Printed and bound in Great Britain by
Mackays of Chatham plc, Kent

CONTENTS

ACKNOWLEDGEMENTS

My grateful thanks go to everyone who helped with the writing of this book – particularly the parents who are quoted talking about their experiences of pregnancy sickness and the many more not mentioned by name.

I am especially grateful to David, Duncan and Alastair Raitt, Linda Carpenter, Caroline Casterton, Christine Hall, Liz McSweeney, Gareth Shannon (SB), Adrian Stoddart, Ann Rowe, Sara Drake, Kathy Levine and MIDIRS, the Royal Society of Medicine, Roy Kelly of Richmond Reference Library, Roy Sherlock and the American Embassy.

FOREWORD

During my first term of office as President of the National Childbirth Trust – wanting to be sure I was in touch with the things women were currently saying were important – I ran discussion groups in eighteen NCT Branches. I simply invited women to talk about their best and worst memories of pregnancy, labour and first postnatal weeks. The subject most frequently mentioned in the whole range of the discussions was sickness in pregnancy, which was discussed spontaneously in seventeen of the eighteen groups. This was not only morning sickness and not just a few weeks of sickness, but all day for five months, or sometimes every day for nine months. One woman's memory of pregnancy was of bending over the loo; others became concerned about whether or not the baby was getting sufficient nourishment, or became housebound and unsociable because they were afraid of being sick when away from home.

This came as a revelation to me. I had enjoyed my pregnancies – never even felt sick – and I was astonished to realise just how common sickness in pregnancy was and how prolonged and how severe the sickness could be. There must be an answer.

In 1988 I appealed to NCT members via New Generation for things that had been found to cure, or even alleviate, sickness in pregnancy. This appeal was repeated in *Chat* magazine thanks to the interest of the editor of the health section. Sixty-eight letters arrived, including some from women for whom the misery had been so great that they had decided not to undergo further pregnancies. I shared all the ideas, publishing lists of what had been found to aggravate the problem and the many and varied things which had been found helpful, with a message about not giving up if the first thing tried didn't work. But I was left with a feeling of disappointment that there was no simple solution which I could pass on in the knowledge that it would provide all sufferers with instant relief.

I was also saddened to learn from those who had suffered that the public at large and the health professionals in particular were not very interested in, or sympathetic about, nausea and vomiting in pregnancy. Perhaps this was because they regarded it as 'normal' and something which would pass, or perhaps they didn't know what to recommend that would definitely help.

Looking back in my files I see I suggested that – as so many women are exceedingly tired around the second to third months of pregnancy and are aware of not functioning properly, in addition to those who are incapacitated by sickness – there was a case for providing a month's maternity leave around that time. There were some clinical trials underway in the late eighties, which I did follow up – but neither the trials nor the popular theories resulted in a sure answer to the problem.

I am therefore delighted that Nicky Wesson has chosen to re-visit the subject in depth. A great many women will be grateful for the existence of this comprehensive study and health professionals will find it a most useful resource.

Eileen Hutton, OBE
President of the NCT 1985–1995
Vice-President of the Community Practitioners'
and Health Visitors' Association

INTRODUCTION

A whole book on morning sickness? If that is your reaction, and I must admit it was mine initially, then you are almost certainly not suffering from it.

While researching this book I had three spells of sickness, the longest lasting 48 hours. They were invaluable in helping me to recall just what unpleasant, embarrassing, humiliating, ignominious symptoms nausea, and particularly vomiting, are; and how unreasonable it is for those caused by pregnancy to carry on week after week, when most illnesses which make you feel sick are over within a couple of days.

It was very important to many of the women that I spoke to that I had suffered pregnancy sickness myself. They felt that unless you have experienced it you cannot really know just how awful it can be. As I asked women at random, many still pregnant, about whether they had morning sickness, I became convinced that the problem is far greater than is generally realised, and that the majority of women do feel really wretched for long stretches of early pregnancy – and some are ill throughout.

Pregnancy is frequently described as 'not being an illness'. This is certainly true in that it is not a disease and there are plenty of people who feel well; perhaps rather fewer who could be described as 'blooming'. However, many expectant mothers feel very ill indeed, and I remember thinking with my first pregnancy that I would have thought I was dying, had I not known I was pregnant.

There are many reasons for the phenomenon of morning sickness being underestimated. Firstly, for most people it occurs in the early weeks of pregnancy – often when they do not want to admit to being pregnant, either because they are fearful that it will not go to full-term or because it has a bearing on their employment, or the time lapse will be too long for their other children to anticipate the birth. For these and other reasons people will try and cope in silence, continuing to work when under other circumstances, such as having a gastric infection, they would be at home in bed.

The very length that pregnancy sickness can last contributes to this – no one would expect to be able to have several weeks off for gastric flu, and unlike a genuine illness it is not seen to come out of the blue but as, to some extent, self-inflicted. Many feel that pregnancy nowadays is considered a matter of choice, that it could be avoided, and so in some way it is a self-indulgent luxury. It can also be hard to admit to pregnancy if you know that colleagues may be jealous, if perhaps they have lost babies or have been unable to conceive. Some women work in a largely male environment where there may be little understanding or tolerance of exclusively female problems. Women who are self-employed or freelance often go to great lengths to conceal difficulties caused by pregnancy. All of these reasons combine to create a conspiracy of silence about the degree of illness it can cause.

Women frequently put other people's needs first. Many women described awful sickness to me but then said, 'I know someone who was much worse.' They seemed to feel that as long as it was not the most severe form they had no right to complain of it. It is almost as if it is regarded as the price you have to pay for having children, and making too much fuss reflects badly on the esteem in which you hold your children.

The disparity between someone who never felt sick and someone who only stops being sick when her baby is born is immense. Pregnancy is a major illness for them; nine months is an appallingly long time to feel ill every single day – always hoping that it might be going to improve. Why do some women have to pay so high a price? It is quite understandable that they resent those who sail through pregnancy, and question whether it is worth it, feeling that their plans of having the number of children that they want is ruined.

As yet there is no answer as to why some suffer more than others, or why some women have it in one pregnancy and not another. Researchers have investigated it in detail: sickness being a clear-cut measurable phenomenon occurring within a specific time span. Their findings are often contradictory so that there appears to be no conclusion that you can safely draw on your chances of getting it again. For example, some may believe it is less likely to occur with older mothers who are having a second or subsequent baby, which might give you hope: others have found the reverse. The stories within this book contain evidence to confound almost every finding.

Another reason that pregnancy sickness fails to be accorded the significance it deserves is the fact that since *Debendox* (*Bendectin*) was taken off the market there is no approved pharmaceutical treatment for it, and when doctors cannot cure you they tend to ignore or dismiss your illness. Moreover, partly through genuine lack of understanding and partly from the old 'What can you expect at your age/in your condition' attitude, doctors often regard pregnancy sickness as to be expected and endured and even as a favourable sign that all is well with the pregnancy.

It is probably true to say that this lack of understanding is in part due to women's reluctance to discuss their symptoms with their doctors. In some of the stories women report either their doctor's failure to take it seriously, or a feeling that there was no point in reporting it as they felt there was little that could be done, unless they were so severely ill that they required rehydration in hospital. Perhaps too, the old psychological slur, that severe pregnancy sickness is all in the mind of hysterical and neurotic women which was believed for so long, makes women loath to approach their doctors. Certainly some of the women I spoke to who had been so ill that they had been admitted to hospital felt that such a charge had been levelled at them – either overtly or tacitly. These women were so very ill that they considered termination of the pregnancy briefly, although they also felt guilty for even thinking of it.

And yes, *I have had it*, almost to the point where I had forgotten that it was not usual to be sick after meals or when cleaning my teeth or coughing.

With my first pregnancy I had a lot of severe abdominal pain which was due to endometriosis and very early heartburn, but I had no sickness until at 10 weeks I was served a scotch egg at a high tea. From that moment I was sick until 20 weeks; my stomach either felt as if I had eaten five school dinners at once, or as if someone had left a bag with bits of the smaller kind of Lego in.

I was haunted by a hideous smell that wasn't there. I spent ages cleaning the kitchen, convinced that there must be a source of the rotten odour. I couldn't believe that no one else could smell it but I eventually had to accept that it didn't exist except in my brain. This apparently unusual symptom was repeated in two other pregnancies, but the smell was different – more 'industrial' and linked with an awful metallic taste in the mouth.

The dog-turd test was diagnostic – I knew I must be pregnant if I had to avert my gaze from pavement excreta. And the cravings varied but have included liquorice sticks, dry roasted peanuts, curry, bananas, crunchy nut corn flakes, boiled sweets and ice cream. I remember a glass of champagne at a wedding going down like battery fluid and, loathing garlic, being deeply suspicious of any salad. It was years before I could face it again. To this day I dislike instant coffee.

I sucked boiled sweets – pear drops last time, solid with alarming colouring – and have been nauseated by exhaust fumes. I have held my breath when passing smokers and been sick in the middle of parties. I have vomited so much that my nose has bled simultaneously – and yet, other people have had it much worse than me and yes, the children are worth it. But it would have been much better *not* to have felt like that. If someone had already compiled this book of suggestions – all of which have helped someone at some time – I might have experienced pregnancy differently. The book's main aim is to let you know that you are not alone. But as inertia and utter exhaustion are two of the symptoms of early pregnancy and it can be hard to find the strength to try out even simple ways of helping yourself to feel better, then this book may be better off in the hands of the pregnant *father*.

As for a one word solution to the problem, I would suggest *zinc*. There are various intriguing clues that add up to it being at least a sizeable part of the answer.

Chapter One

THE HISTORY OF MORNING SICKNESS

Pregnancy sickness has been with us for a long time. The earliest records come from a papyrus which is dated two thousand years BC and it was referred to by Hippocrates. The most detailed of the early descriptions come from Soranus who practised medicine in Rome in the first half of the second century AD. His work on obstetrics and gynaecology lasted through various translations, and his views and practices survived right through the Middle Ages to the sixteenth century.

It was further translated by Temkin (1956) who found that Soranus described how the sickness of pregnancy sets in around the 40th day and lasts for about four months. He stated that 'if the fetus is male, its movements will be both slower and more sluggish, while the gravida (mother) too, moves with little ease and has a stronger inclination to vomiting'. He also says: 'Some women are also affected with vomiting at intervals or at each meal, or with a feeling of weariness, dizziness, headache, discomfort together with an abundance of raw humours, pallor, the appearance of under nourishment and constipation. Some also have gastric distension or pain in the thorax. The same persons sometimes also show very slight fever and swelling up at the breasts and some display jaundice.'

Soranus had a very detailed list of recommendations and remedies, some of which may well be worth trying today. These included fasting for a day and being rubbed with ointment. After the fast the expectant mother was supposed to start by eating a soft-boiled egg, porridge and then lean fowl. She should then have a hot bath and take a little weak wine. At first she should take exercise passively as in a sedan chair, working up gradually to dancing and punching a leather bag. She should be massaged daily and then reduce the daily bath to one every two to three days. Her stomach should be bound with wool soaked in the oil of unripe olives, and an upset stomach should be treated with oil of roses, quinces, myrtle, mastic and spikenard (essential oils of most of these are still available today). In the case of vomiting she should put plasters of dry date boiled in tart wine or diluted vinegar onto the stomach – these could be made more powerful by the addition of moist or dry alum, aloe, mastic, roses, saffron, bloom of the wild vine, pomegranate peel, omphakion, oak gall, hypnocist, acacia or the finest meal of barley.

The next known reference to morning sickness and *hyperemesis gravidarum* (severe pregnancy sickness) is from a book written by Jacques Guillemeau (1612), called *Childbirth or the Happy Deliverie of Women*. Guillemeau suggested that pregnancy sickness was caused by 'the abundance of humours gathered together in the stomach'. Nicholas Culpepper (1651) also mentions 'diverse longings and continual vomiting' in his *Directory for Midwives* and describes them as being as among the earliest signs of pregnancy.

John Burton (1751) of Wakefield and York describes pregnancy sickness as being caused 'solely from the stoppage of the menstrual flux'. William Smellie (1779) in Book II of his *Treatise on the Theory and Practice of Midwifery* observed that 'the first complaint attending pregnancy is the nausea and vomiting which in some women begins soon after conception and frequently continues till the end of the fourth month. Most women are troubled with this symptom more or less, particularly vomiting in the morning. Some who have no such complaint in one pregnancy shall be violently attacked with it in another and in a few it prevails during the whole time of uterine gestation.' He thought it was caused by 'stretching fullness of the vessels' and considered that it would be improved by bleeding and opening medicines and emollient glysters to relieve costiveness (constipation).

Fox (1834), who considered nausea and vomiting almost inevitable in pregnancy and observed that it generally decreased at about the time fetal movements could be felt, recommended effervescent soda and water several times a day. Persistent sufferers were recommended to apply linen soaked in laudanum to the stomach together with 8–10 leeches. He also appreciated, perhaps more helpfully, that frequent resting, lying down, helped too.

There is no apparent recognition of the fact that the severest form of pregnancy sickness – *hyperemesis gravidarum*, could actually be fatal, until the late eighteenth century, when Vaughan (1789) described having saved a woman's life by feeding her rectally. A classic description of *hyperemesis gravidarum* leading to death was given by Paul DuBois (1852), who wrote of women suffering from constant vomiting, frequent dribbling of saliva, and considerable emaciation, while their urine became scanty and highly coloured and their pulse rate increased. Later on, he claimed, their vomiting became still more pronounced and their breath smelled peculiarly acid and fetid. Their pulse increased in frequency and they might have a slight rise in temperature. Finally, the women appeared to get better for a short time and stop vomiting for a while before becoming delirious and dying in coma or while having convulsions.

Fortunately, medical treatment means that no one need die in this way these days, but at the time DuBois was writing the only treatment was to terminate the pregnancy. Debate raged as to whether this would improve the condition or make it worse. DuBois believed it was useful, and used the example of ten of his patients who died from pernicious vomiting as it was then known: however, of the four in whom abortion was induced, only one survived.

Death from pregnancy sickness was recorded as recently as 1939 (Sheehan, 1939) and in fact Charlotte Brontë died from it in 1855. The description of her illness by Mrs Gaskell and the letters she wrote to her friends graphically convey her suffering. Her description of her illness parallels that of DuBois with startling accuracy.

Ann Dally (1982), in her book *Inventing Motherhood* details Charlotte Brontë's illness:

... in November 1854, just over three months after her returning from a honeymoon in Ireland, Charlotte developed a cold, which lingered, but does not seem to have been serious. In the new year she was attacked by new sensations of perpetual nausea and ever-recurring faintness. Charlotte wrote on January 19th to her friend Ellen Nassey: 'My health has been really very good since my return from Ireland till about ten days ago, when the stomach seemed quite suddenly to lose its tone – indigestion and continual faint sickness have been my portion ever since.' She seems to associate this with her pregnancy for she continues, 'Don't conjecture, dear Nell, for it is too soon yet though I certainly never before felt as I have done lately.' Her husband called in Dr. MacTurk from Bradford, who 'assigned a natural cause for her miserable indisposition'. Martha, the maid, tenderly waited on her mistress, and from time to time tried to cheer her with the thought of the baby that was coming. 'I dare say I shall be glad sometime' she would say 'but I am so ill, so weary . . .' Then she took to her bed, too weak to sit up. Some time in February, she wrote to Amelia Taylor: 'Let me speak the plain truth – my sufferings are very great – my nights indescribable – sickness with scarce a reprieve – I strain until what I vomit is mixed with blood.' Mrs. Gaskell tells us: 'About the third week in March there was a change; a low wandering delirium came on; and in it she begged constantly for food and even for stimulants. She swallowed eagerly now; but it was too late.' On March 31st she died.

In the twentieth century, effective treatment has been made available so that women no longer die from pregnancy sickness although it may still be very severe and require admission to hospital. However, treatment itself has advanced and retreated with the notorious drug treatment *Thalidomide*, and later *Debendox*.

Thalidomide was developed in the 1950s by a German company. Sold as a sedative, it was marketed as being entirely safe and without side effects. In fact there was little legislation at the time to ensure that these claims were true; it had not been tested for safety on animals and only crudely tested on humans. Its safety in pregnancy was unproven but it was popularly prescribed because of the claims made for it. It was first used in 1958. By 1961 reports began to come in linking its use in early pregnancy with severe limb defects in newborn babies. By this time the drug had been marketed world-wide and the consequences were disastrous. Over 10,000 babies were born with severe deformities, having legs or arms missing or partly missing. The drug was so teratogenic (Priest, 1990) that one pill taken between the 27th and 33rd day of pregnancy would be almost 100% certain to cause deformity in the fetus. Eventually the link became indisputable and the drug was banned. Since then doctors and mothers have been very cautious about prescribing or taking medication in pregnancy, in particular during the first fourteen weeks when the baby is forming.

This new caution affected the prescriptions of *Debendox*, an anti-nausea drug which was first used in 1964. It was said to be highly successful but was eventually removed from sale in 1983 because 250 people sued the company for its having allegedly caused birth defects in their children. By this time it had been used by 33 million women world-wide without there having been any evidence of its causing defects. However, the company wished to avoid further lawsuits – one mother sued for $75 million – and the drug was no longer available to relieve pregnancy sickness despite being, as described by Kousen (1993), an editor of *Teratology*, 'the most famous tortogen/litogen and the best studied human non-teratogen'.

Drug treatments are currently available but the legacy of *Thalidomide* means that they are only prescribed for the severest forms of pregnancy sickness where there is a risk to the health of the mother.

For the all too common but lesser degree of sickness, the types of remedy available are not much more developed than those suggested by Soranus almost two thousand years ago.

(For further details of the history of morning sickness see Chapter Six.)

Chapter Two

WHO GETS MORNING SICKNESS?

Some nausea and vomiting is so common as to be described as normal. Beverley O'Brien (O'Brien & Naber, 1995) recognises that 70–90% of all pregnant women experience some nausea while 50% vomit at least once. There is plenty of research on the subject and many people have tried to determine what causes it, who is most likely to suffer from it and why this should be. Despite this research, no firm conclusions can be drawn, particularly as the research findings are in conflict or, as O'Brien puts it, 'some investigators reported a positive association between symptoms and a particular variable, whereas others failed to support that association or even find a negative association'. For example, some found that older women were more likely to suffer – others found that it was more likely in younger women.

The type of variables investigated have included:

- the number of children a woman has
- her level of education
- her weight
- her personality factors
- her smoking habits
- the sex of the baby
- the birthweight of the baby
- the race of mother and baby
- whether the baby was conceived before marriage
- if the mother was going out to work or a housewife

The differing results may be due in part to the fact that women are more likely to recall symptoms if they are asked about them at the time they have them, rather than later. Some of the ways of assessing the severity of symptoms differed too. In some studies women were included if they had mild nausea, while others were only included if they had actually vomited. In some, their condition was assessed by their carers, whereas in others, the women's own views of how they felt were regarded as being most significant.

Unsurprisingly, women who were unable to alter their working conditions, especially those working in fast food outlets, were found to be most likely to suffer. O'Brien also found some evidence to suggest that oestrogen production and metabolism are altered by a woman's first full-term pregnancy, so that the amount of free oestriol (and consequent nausea and vomiting) is lower in subsequent pregnancies. She also found that smokers experience less nausea, although smoking also reduces fertility and birthweight. This may be because it has an effect on the endocrine system, or because smoking notoriously blunts the senses of taste and smell which are significantly involved in nausea and vomiting (see Chapter Three). Women who are sick when they take the contraceptive pill, or who are travel sick or sick with migraines are more likely to get pregnancy sickness.

O'Brien found that there does seem to be a weak but significant increase in suffering with those women who are pregnant with girls (although other researchers have not found this to be so). It is true that the amniotic fluid surrounding female fetuses contains higher concentrations of human chorionic gonadotrophin than that around males, but this is not a strong enough basis on which to make a correct assumption about the sex of your child.

However, the cause remains unexplained and it is not possible to predict who will suffer most. Women whose vomiting becomes so severe as to warrant admission to hospital, through being a captive study sample as well as presenting with a very distressing condition, have exercised researchers still further and there is a wealth of research which has considered the cause and treatment of their condition, known as *hyperemesis gravidarum* (excessive pregnancy sickness). This is considered in Chapter Four.

Clearly it is important to ascertain that such a drastic symptom is caused purely by pregnancy. Alison Archibald's story (p. 34) shows that it is quite possible to attribute pregnancy sickness to another cause, and while in her case this did no harm, it is possible for a serious illness to be missed if it is dismissed as being due to pregnancy alone. The list of differential diagnoses, or things that might cause sickness other than pregnancy include:

Gastro-intestinal and hepatobiliary causes:
Peptic disorders
Diaphragmatic hernia
Pyelitis
Hepatitis
Biliary tract disease
Pancreatitis

Appendicitis
Inflammatory or obstructive bowel disease
Genito-urinary infection
Pyelonephritis
Uraemia
Twisted ovarian cyst
Red degeneration of fibroids

Miscellaneous
Drug toxicity
Diabetic ketosis
Hyperthyroidism
Central nervous system lesions
Vestibular disorders and others including food poisoning, viruses and
  urinary tract infection

· *Lesley* ·

*It wasn't a problem. I went off tea with number five – that's all. That was
a nuisance because of the social implications: sitting down to a glass of
water just isn't the same.*

*I did want Marmite – they used to laugh at me at work because I
asked to have a cheese and marmite roll but there had to be more
Marmite than cheese.*

*One long-lasting benefit is that now I get a cup of tea in bed in the
morning. We used to take it in turns but since I was pregnant Tony
always brings it to me.*

· *Janice Coulson* ·

*The first time I was pregnant, it was not too bad, it got worse with subse-
quent pregnancies.*

*My first pregnancy was much wanted and before I became pregnant
I often used to wonder while waiting for a period, how I would feel if I
was pregnant – could I be this time? The actual weekend before it was
confirmed I was doing a lot of work and Mike kept bringing me cups of
coffee which tasted horrible. I did wonder if it was the coffee or whether I
might be pregnant – three days later I knew I was.*

*I remember looking at my face in the mirror and it no longer seemed
puffy as it did at the start of a period, so I still seemed to be following my
cycle – two weeks later I was a bit tired but by the time I was six weeks I
was full scale nauseated and so hungry.*

I did not normally have breakfast and often skipped lunch. After the nausea started I used to have breakfast – cornflakes usually, nothing too sweet, and then by 11 o'clock I would be cruising past the bakery in Richmond thinking, 'No I mustn't, yes I must!' I'd go in to get two white rolls with huge chunks of cheese. I had a passion for white bread, I couldn't tolerate brown, it seemed too sweet.

By the seventh week onwards I was never sick but if I got hungry I started to get nauseated. I remember being offered a very strong cup of tea in someone's house but I could only take a sip because it made me feel sick. I felt iffy until 10 weeks and had to eat to stop the nausea.

At 10 weeks we went on holiday to Rhodes. I felt very sick being driven to the airport in the back of a taxi. While we were away, I got so hungry we would have to go out foraging at eleven o'clock at night. I put on a stone in the first twelve weeks of pregnancy.

When we got back I was exactly 12 weeks and felt a lot better, not too sick at all. The only time I was sick was when I was 38 weeks pregnant. I had a corned beef sandwich with my elderly relations one afternoon. At the time I was trying to get a grip on the bladder problems of late pregnancy and was trying to train myself out of running to the loo all the time. That night I vomited all night and went up to the hospital in the morning because I had a temperature and was starting to get pains in my back. It turned out that I had both a urine and kidney infection which I had not really been aware of – I attributed the vomiting to the sandwich.

I did find that my tastes had changed – I wanted to eat beef crisps which I wouldn't normally choose. They livened up my mouth and zapped my taste buds and took away that constant horrible taste.

The next full-term pregnancy went according to the same sort of pattern – needing something to eat to quell the nausea. I was about a stone heavier at the start of this pregnancy but put on 9lb less so that I ended up at the same weight at the end of both pregnancies. My body seemed to adjust itself.

The difference when I was expecting Ralph though was that I was able to sleep in the afternoon while Alice had a nap. We were between two houses at the time and had a lot of decorating to do but being able to sleep made a lot of difference. I felt a lot more sick when tired – I did gag a few times but was never actually sick.

The next two pregnancies ended in miscarriage. One at eighteen weeks, I had felt really dreadful. I was still breast feeding until I was 12 weeks, Alice was four and Ralph 20 months and he wore me out. I only felt better at 16 weeks – in the last week I felt great. It was good because the nausea seemed to be over but it turned out that the baby, a boy, had died.

I had felt so bad that although I was devastated at losing the baby, I was really relieved not to be pregnant any more. It balanced out in some way.

Exactly one year to the day I was pregnant again – with these two I felt nauseous even before I had missed a period. This time I felt absolutely lousy – draggingly nauseated. It was very wearing – it helped to eat some-

*thing but the effect wore off after half an hour. The timing meant that I
was feeling ill all through the Christmas parties, nativity plays and
Christmas dinner. I just dragged round them all feeling awful. I lost the
baby at 14 weeks ...*

Two effects of the nausea linger – one is Alice's Golden Sound toy of
Beauty and the Beast: *although it is three or four years later, if she touches the magic mirror which makes a crackly sound I still feel sick. Also we
have stretch couch covers in a bright jade green. Although I've got over it
now, they used to make me feel nauseated every time I looked at them
even though I was no longer pregnant.*

If you are being sick several times a day you could become dehydrated; you should see your GP or midwife. However, it can be useful
to know the signs that warrant further attention in case you do not get
it from your primary carer.

Clinical signs of dehydration:
- Weight loss
- Rising pulse rate (120 beats per minute and above)
- Falling blood pressure (lower reading (diastolic) – 50 and below)
- Dry and furry tongue
- Loss of skin elasticity (if you pinch your skin, it only returns to
  normal gradually)
- Your breath will smell ketotic (it smells of nail varnish or pear drops
  – ask someone else to tell you)
- You will not urinate very often, and when you do, your urine will be
  dark yellow and there will not be much of it.

If you have any of these symptoms while you are being sick
frequently, you need to get medical help. You should get help too if the
physical strain of vomiting is causing premature contractions or bleeding. If you fail to get it from your GP, contact your midwife or consultant obstetrician.

One director of midwifery stressed the importance of getting help if
vomiting is causing dehydration. She says that GPs vary as to how
sympathetically they regard the condition – and feels that it is very
important that it is not ignored. She recommends that if your doctor
does not take it seriously or you do not have a midwife you should go
direct to the maternity unit with which you are booked, or if not yet
booked, go straight to the Accident & Emergency department which
will ensure that you get help. She feels that women with *hyperemesis
gravidarum* in the very early stages of pregnancy should be admitted
to the maternity wards rather than gynaecology to provide an encouraging atmosphere.

There are also some conditions of pregnancy which can make nausea and vomiting worse. None are particularly common but should be considered if you are being very sick. They are:

- Hydatidiform mole
- Twin/multiple pregnancy
- Pregnancy induced hypertension
- Hydramnios
- Placental abruption

Hydatidiform mole or molar pregnancy

This is a rare complication of pregnancy only found in 1 in 2,000 pregnancies in the UK but much more common in Russia, Mexico, the Philippines, and Formosa where the incidence is 1 in 120 pregnancies.

The placental tissue develops in the same way that it does in a potential miscarriage as a blighted ovum, where part of the pregnancy cells grow in the absence of a fetus. In this case the chorionic villi develop unusually, so that they produce large quantities of the hormone human chorionic gonadotrophin (*HCG*), thus maintaining the pregnancy and giving a very positive pregnancy test reading. It is usually described as looking like a bunch of tiny grapes which are actually cysts. The extremely high levels of *HCG* cause considerable pregnancy sickness, which together with the abdominal swelling mean that the diagnosis should be considered.

You should seek help if you have:

- severe sickness
- are much bigger than expected for your dates
- have intermittent bleeding, particularly if you are passing little cysts.

Other possible indications of a molar pregnancy may include the following:

- your blood pressure is raised early in pregnancy
- you have protein in your urine at an early stage of pregnancy
- you are bleeding by 12 weeks
- you are anaemic
- you have pain in the pelvis
- no heart beat or baby can be found on ultrasound.

Hospital treatment is needed in order to remove the mole, and you should undergo careful monitoring of blood and urine samples for the next two years as there is a very small chance that any remaining chorionic villi may have become malignant. (See Case History p. 23.)

Twin/multiple pregnancy

It seems logical that being pregnant with two or more babies would make you more sick, although this is not invariably so. (See Case Histories pp.25 and 45.)

Pregnancy-induced hypertension

Although not one of the commonly recognised symptoms of PET (*pre-eclamptic toxaemia*), vomiting in the second half of pregnancy may be caused by raised blood pressure. This may be due to cerebral oedema (swelling of the brain) or related to pain from under the ribs as a result of haemorrhage around the liver. It is important to be aware of it as a possibility because PET can start suddenly and if left untreated it can be fatal. You should always contact your midwife or doctor if you have any of these symptoms, even without vomiting:

- severe headaches which cannot be relieved by painkillers
- visual disturbances, e.g. seeing flashing lights
- abdominal pain
- considerable swelling

It is to detect PET that your blood pressure reading is taken at each antenatal check.

Hydramnios

This is when you have an excess of amniotic fluid: the increased size of your uterus may give rise to nausea and heartburn.

Placental abruption

If some of the placenta peels away from your uterus before birth it will result in bleeding, either from the vagina or internally, and shock. It is a rare complication of pregnancy, likely to result in your abdomen becoming rock-hard due to internal bleeding, and giving rise to severe pain which might make you feel sick. *In such circumstances you should go to hospital immediately.*

· *Caroline* ·

With my first pregnancy I miscarried after 10 weeks and I learned just how common this is. It was pronounced a 'normal' miscarriage and so I was told I could try to conceive again when I felt emotionally ready as there were no physical implications.

I waited 4 months before I found I had became pregnant again, confirmed by a home test. I was happy but anxious and tried to register with my GP as soon as possible, but couldn't get an appointment until I was 8 weeks. I had started to feel increasingly sick all day, very emotional and tired, but my doctor reassured me this was nothing to be concerned about even though I seemed to be 'big for dates', as this could be twins. At 10 weeks I started bleeding so I went back to my doctor (a different one as my original doctor had no spaces available) who recommended me for a scan. I went to casualty and had to wait, as no appointment could be made, but luckily the registrar was able to give a vaginal scan where, to my relief, a heartbeat was identified. She suggested I have a full ultrasound within a week but I had to wait another 4 weeks. I felt very, very sick and nothing made any difference: eating or not eating, relaxing or keeping busy, it was always the same. I felt increasingly ill but it was difficult to get my doctor to respond to the urgency I felt. By the time the ultrasound appointment arrived my abdomen was very distended. I was still bleeding, though less so, and I couldn't sleep due to abdominal pain. I had a strange taste in my mouth and felt emotionally and physically exhausted. My GP told me not to be concerned as everybody experiences pregnancy so individually. Looking back now I realise I was very ill.

My husband came with me for the scan. The radiographer kept quiet without answering our questions. Eventually we were told the pregnancy was not viable and that it was a molar pregnancy with cysts in the womb. I also had numerous ovarian cysts. We were left alone while a doctor was called, both of us feeling shocked and sad. I was taken to the ward straight away and a doctor came to tell me about the risks of a molar pregnancy, how it could develop into cancer, and about the risks of having an anaesthetic for the evacuation that was urgently needed. She stressed the risks and I came home very upset and scared, concerned for my wellbeing and anxious as to the implications.

The next morning I was admitted to hospital and came home that evening, That was it, without any further explanation despite all my questions. There was no back-up counselling, just a review appointment and scan in two weeks. I was told I could go back to work within a few days but I ended up taking two weeks off.

Having a medical background I was determined to find out more but there wasn't much at the library, only that the 'risk of cancer' kept cropping up.

At the review the ovarian cysts were found up under my diaphragm but I was told they would regress naturally as the pregnancy hormone levels decreased. The placental cysts had been successfully evacuated together with the fetus which had developed as a result of the partial molar pregnancy and as a result had not survived.

The follow-up consisted of weekly visits for blood samples which were sent to Charing Cross Hospital together with a urine sample. It took six

months for my HCG level to return to normal which means a follow up
for two years of monthly urine samples to ensure there are no repercus-
sions (it is less than this if the levels return to normal quicker).

One of the senior members at Charing Cross finally managed to give
me an explanation as to what a molar or partial molar pregnancy means.
Apparently it is a similar mechanism to having twins, but instead of four
sets of chromosomes there are only three, hence the fetus. The other one
somehow causes the placenta to keep producing the HCG after the three
month period when this task should shift to the ovaries and reduce the
HCG level. It is this increase in production of HCG which causes excessive
sickness and ovarian cysts, plus the development of placental cysts which
override any developing fetus. The evacuation is to ensure all tissue is
cleared and the tests determine if the remaining chromosome reactivates
itself in which case it could develop into cancer. Once the HCG level is
normal there is a six month wait before conceiving again with a 1 in 75
risk of recurrence, although this is less for a partial molar.

In my quest for answers I have seen both an osteopath and homeopath
who identified some imbalances and have been incredibly helpful. I tried a
de-tox diet for a week and now, seven months later, I am feeling healthier
than I have for a long time. My husband, too, feels more confident. I think
sometimes we forget that it is not just women who feel the shock.

Passing the due date was a milestone. It's as if the body has a cycle of
its own which is followed, even if the pregnancy is lost, and it is since that
time that, physically and emotionally, I have felt stronger. I feel anxious
about the future but am determined to be positive, and I feel lucky that I
have such a wonderful relationship with my husband, as we have been
through this together, which has made an enormous difference.

· *Caroline Davis* ·

I think the first pregnancy was my worst because it went on longer. I had
had two miscarriages prior to that when I had been sick, and then at eight
weeks, both times, it suddenly stopped and then I miscarried. My doctors
suggested that I have hormone injections to prevent another miscarriage,
saying it wouldn't do any harm. The hospital subsequently put the severity
of my symptoms down to that decision. Sickness that time continued until
I was seven months pregnant. It was so bad, that by the time I was just
seven-and-a-half weeks pregnant I had lost a stone-and-a-half. The sickness lasted all day; if I was awake I felt awful, there was no relief. I lost
count of the number of times that I was sick during the day: eventually I
did all the actions without there even being bile, that had long since gone!

I was admitted to hospital and found the rehydration wonderful. They
put a drip up straightaway as I think my doctor had sent a letter with me
and they took it seriously. The sensation of the rehydration was wonder-

ful – within an hour I could feel the water coming back into me and I could feel moisture in my mouth and nose again. At least that time I only had myself to look after. I worked for a bank in Birmingham and they were very good about it; I had ten weeks off work altogether. I worked up until 28 weeks and then stopped as soon as I could. I was still being sick – I used to get to work and make straight for the loo, but I felt guilty about taking so much time off, and as the job was one I had created I felt I needed to hand it over to someone else and explain it properly.

With my second daughter it was not as bad, it didn't last as long, but I was desperate for a third baby. Each time, I started being sick before my period was due. Ginger and Marmite helped, but only until I was too sick to face them.

With my third child, I had to be admitted again when I was seven weeks pregnant. My own doctor, once I saw him, was very good, he had me admitted at once. I originally spoke to one of the other doctors who is rather male-oriented and not very sympathetic to women's problems. He just said, 'You will suffer, just drink flat Coke and it will go away'. At the hospital they mentioned that such extreme sickness could be due to multiple pregnancy, but I just laughed it off. The next morning they took me for a scan to make sure that the sickness was caused by pregnancy as I had felt so awful that I hadn't done a test. I was so weak by then that it took two people to support me in order for me to stand up, and they took me for the scan in a wheelchair. I remember thinking that I hoped I was pregnant. After the first scan they said they wanted to do an internal one to get some more detail and I started to get concerned. Then they said 'We weren't sure at first but we are now – you are expecting twins!' The rush of adrenaline made me feel better for half-an-hour, but after that the sickness was back again.

I was on the drip for about a week – I had it with me at all times, and could get up to go to the loo. For the first two days though I could hear people talking and talking about me, but I was too ill to respond. I slept for two days and then gradually got better. In fact I did manage to eat a bit there because the food arrived ready-cooked. Later, when I could smell food cooking but it was a while before it appeared, I couldn't eat it when it arrived. I hated all kitchen smells and used to spray a perfume around to try and get rid of them – our cupboards smelled awful! That perfume makes me feel ill even now.

I came out of hospital and then, at nine weeks, I couldn't see how I was going to manage. I even thought about an abortion (although I would never have one) just because I felt so awful. In fact I went to stay with my parents who luckily live nearby. I lived with them for six weeks until it started to improve. I couldn't do anything for my children – I couldn't tie a dress bow or do up their shoes, and my parents did it all for me. My mother used to come in with water and say, 'You must drink.' I took it, but it felt like a ton weight in my stomach.

It did start to get better at thirteen weeks and, once I could eat, I craved green vegetables and all sorts of healthy foods. I caught up and gained weight so that by 38 weeks I was begging them to induce me because I was so huge. Eventually they did, because the scan showed that the head circumferences had not grown in the last week. My babies weighed 6lb 8 oz and 5lb 4 oz although they were two weeks early!

You do forget, and can even be grateful, that pregnancy sickness means that you are not likely to miscarry. But I remember thinking, when the twins were six months old, that coping with them and a two-and-a-half year old and a four year old was a doddle compared with pregnancy.

Chapter Three

How it may affect you

· *The physical effects* ·

If you are reading this book, the chances are that you will have all too good an idea of the way morning sickness can make you feel. However, symptoms do vary from person to person and may be different from one pregnancy to the next or even during the course of pregnancy. Forewarned is not necessarily fore-armed in this case, but it can be helpful to know that some of the more eccentric manifestations are normal.

Morning sickness is to be expected in that the majority of pregnant women suffer either from nausea or vomiting or both. Although not limited to the morning, or just to the first 14 weeks, it is far from unusual, although there are plenty of mothers around who claim never to have experienced it, or only felt a twinge 'for half an hour, on two evenings'.

Morning sickness is clearly linked to the digestive system but it can affect all the senses – smell in particular, but also taste and touch. Some women find nausea induced by things that they see and handle and even altering position or standing for a long time makes some people sick. There seems to be a strong link with the awful tiredness of early pregnancy too, so that far from being radiant, most women feel pretty dreadful in the early weeks.

Estimates of the percentage of women who are affected by nausea and vomiting vary, but some idea is given by two large-scale studies, each of which reflected the experiences of 1000 women. A particularly informative study which was prospective, i.e. recruited women before pregnancy and followed them through, is the Avon (1992) 'Children of the Nineties' which will involve 15,000 women altogether. The first thousand women were asked about their early pregnancy when they reached eighteen weeks. The results showed that 67% had felt nausea and 41% had vomited while 64% felt less active.

The other study, done at St George's Hospital in London found that 85% experienced nausea, 70% having had it every day, while 52% had vomited, 40% of them daily (Whitehead *et al.*, 1992). These women completed their questionnaires earlier in pregnancy, at 15 weeks on average, which may explain why the figures show that more women suffered from the symptoms. Most people are glad to forget about nausea and vomiting, when and if it subsides.

This study also showed that a third of the mothers had started to feel ill within four weeks of their last period, while three quarters had started within six weeks. It seems that the sooner you start, the more likely you are to have daily nausea and/or vomiting. Less than half found that their symptoms were limited to the morning.

The nausea of pregnancy can vary from slight to extreme and alter daily in the time it lasts and its severity. Barbara Pickard (1984) says that most women find it worst on an empty stomach: they start by retching first thing in the morning which is doubtless the origin of the concept of morning sickness. They may also retch before eating or vomit during or after meals. Women often feel like eating immediately after being sick and then feel better, only for the symptoms to return gradually.

The nature of pregnancy sickness can be different from being sick ordinarily. Vomiting may occur without warning and some women report it as being easier than vomiting through illness. Often vomiting relieves the nausea so that being sick is preferable to feeling continually nauseous. However, it can be truly wretched and leave you with sore throat, aching ribs and stomach muscles, congested face with running eyes and nose. Indeed it can easily provoke nose bleeds which are more common in pregnancy, and leave your head aching. Allied symptoms may include cramps, intense hunger, the metallic taste in the mouth, excessive salivation, a terrific thirst and a feeling of weakness and extreme tiredness. You may also lose a lot of weight – or gain it if eating is the only thing that staves off nausea. Altogether, it is hardly surprising if a lack of excitement about pregnancy can be included in the list of symptoms.

· *Symptoms associated with pregnancy* · *and morning sickness*

Hunger

You may find yourself intensely hungry, so that you feel you have to eat immediately, and when you do it may either keep the nausea off for a while or you may be sick straightaway. (See Case History p. 33.)

Cravings

The desire to eat a particular food is sometimes overwhelming. The food is often something that you do not normally like. It seems likely that this is your body demanding something that you are lacking, whether it is glucose or a trace element or mineral.

Pica

This is the desire to eat something inedible, formerly a well-recognised symptom of pregnancy. It is much less frequently recorded now, probably because women's diets are now more diverse and better balanced. However, the St George's study found that nearly half of the women had food cravings for one particular thing. . . . 'Over half the women (52%) with nausea found that eating helped to ease nausea, but only a third with vomiting found it improved the symptoms. Women who developed food cravings were more likely to experience nausea.'

Food aversion

As well as craving certain foods, many women experience aversion to things that they have previously enjoyed. Coffee and alcohol are common examples. It has been argued that this is due to the action of hormones on a part of the brain known as the area postema which is known as the chemoreceptor trigger zone, involved with vomiting, and also with taste aversions (Whitehead *et al.*, 1992). More simply, it may be that there is a protective function – that you 'go off' foods and drink that would harm your developing baby. (For more about food cravings and aversions see p. 37.)

Metallic taste

This is the unpleasant coppery taste which can be present even in the early weeks. Once described as being like sucking old pennies, it can spoil the taste of food and this is described as being troublesome for those who suffered moderate to severe symptoms in a study that described the effects of nausea and vomiting during pregnancy on the quality of life (O'Brien & Naber, 1995). One of the participants is quoted as having 'a real metallic taste in her mouth that was continuously present, thus making even drinking water very unpleasant' (O'Brien & Zhou, 1992). (See Case Histories pp. 37, 45 and 47.)

Heartburn

Described as a 'searing pain at bottom of windpipe', (Winkler, 1985) heartburn is one of the miseries of pregnancy that is normally associated with the later stages, when it is suggested that the cause is mechanical as a result of the uterus expanding and pushing upwards. However, some mothers get it really early in pregnancy, suggesting a hormonal cause. Progesterone, which has a softening effect on the tissues, and is produced in pregnancy to maintain the pregnancy and help develop the uterus, relaxes the valve at the upper end of the stomach. This means that stomach acid can be forced up into the oesophagus, to a part of the tube where it never normally reaches, and which is not immune to the effects of acid, unlike the stomach. This burns the tissues, causing inflammation. Later on the expansion of the ribs can result in a further opening of the valve so that acid may pass up more easily. In this situation, lying down or bending down can made the heartburn worse. (See Case History p. 33.)

Burping

Excess gas can form in the stomach and give rise to an unpleasant sensation of fullness and nausea. Although it has been suggested that this is due to swallowing air, (Bourne, 1984) it seems to develop naturally. Burping may occur frequently and will relieve the nausea at least temporarily. However, if heartburn is also causing problems, the relief of nausea may well be accompanied by a surge of heartburn as stomach acids are pushed into the oesophagus with the air, causing it to become more inflamed.

Excessive salivation

Technically known as *ptyalism*, this is when saliva output is so increased that it becomes impossible to swallow it, and it has to be spat out into a handkerchief. (See Case History p. 42.)

Smell

As well as experiencing alterations in taste, you may find that your sense of smell is impaired too. You may find that pleasant smells become obnoxious, particularly cooking and food smells, but also perfumes or soaps. More understandably, exhaust fumes or cigarette smoke may seem extra unpleasant. There could be a protective purpose for this but it can make it particularly difficult if you are unable to avoid them. An American researcher, Donna Van Lier, and others (1993) discovered that the smells that were least appreciated by pregnant women were onions, perfume, trash cans, diaper pails (nappy buckets), vehicle exhaust and cigarette smoke. Toothpaste has also been mentioned (Korte, 1995; Anderson, 1994). Eileen Hutton (1988), in a survey of 68 mothers who had experienced pregnancy sickness, found that the smells that exacerbated symptoms were cooking, strong perfumes, smoking, anything commonly regarded as 'a bad smell', and bleach. (See Case Histories pp. 37 and 47.)

Visual

As in non-pregnancy sickness, truly unpleasant sights can make you vomit spontaneously, or at least feel very queasy. In pregnancy sickness, the threshold may be lowered so that everyday things can produce the same reaction. I remember being offered a biscuit by a woman who took the lid off the tin and held it out at arm's length and with her head averted. Curiously she wasn't sure at that stage whether or not she was pregnant.

Anything fairly obnoxious in normal circumstances, such as changing nappies, may become more unpleasant. Some women even find that feeding toddlers can become impossibly nauseating.

Motion or travel sickness

This can be exacerbated in pregnancy so that it may become marked in women who never normally get it. Those who are prone to travel sickness are unfortunately more likely than most to suffer from pregnancy sickness generally, but particularly while travelling by car, boat or plane. (See Case History p. 34.)

Touch

Even touch can become nauseating. One woman in Beverley O'Brien's study of the effect of nausea and vomiting on the quality of women's lives said 'any sort of movement, such as my husband sitting on the bed, or twisting and turning in bed at night would make me very nauseated. If my son wanted to come and climb all over me, which he is used to doing, that would make me very nauseated' (O'Brien & Naber, 1995). Feeling nauseous if anyone touches you can contribute to some of the difficulties in relationships, which are not uncommon in early pregnancy.

Tiredness or fatigue

Extreme tiredness or lethargy is very common in early pregnancy. It can be almost completely overwhelming and come as a considerable shock. If you have never been pregnant, it is probably very difficult to understand how tiring this stage can be. It could be compared to the exhaustion of serious illness. There may be a link between pregnancy sickness and tiredness. Certainly some researchers have found that if you have a severe form of one symptom, you are more likely to experience the other as well. However, it is not possible to say that one causes the other, although it may be that the stimulus is the same for both. Many women have found that resting with their feet up has helped improve their symptoms of nausea or vomiting.

Donna Van Lier in her study with Manteuffel and Dilorio (1993), on nausea and fatigue during early pregnancy, examined 65 women who were less than 16 weeks pregnant. She asked women how tired they felt using a descriptive scale ranging from '– extremely peppy(!)' (1) to '– ready to drop' (10). As many as 88% of the women described themselves as suffering from nausea and exactly the same percentage suffered from tiredness, averaging level 6 – 'slightly pooped' (this is an American study). Those who suffered the highest levels of nausea experienced the most fatigue. Although this study was too small to generalise about, it was clear that in some women, fatigue increased nausea and in others it was the other way around.

A larger study by O'Brien & Naber (1995) found that recumbent rest was the second most valuable way of reducing nausea and vomiting (25%): eating was the first (52.8%). They quote one woman as saying 'I would go in my room and shut the door and ask that nobody would come in. I didn't want to talk to anybody, I didn't want to smell the odors of anything; I didn't want anybody bumping my mattress. If I could just sit and be as still as I could and try and sleep. I tried to sleep so much, because at least then I didn't feel my stomach turn.'

Unfortunately, even if you know that resting will help reduce nausea and vomiting, it can be really difficult to get or take time off, especially as these symptoms are likely to occur at a time when you may not want to make your pregnancy public. (See Case History below.)

Coughing

This is not currently recognised as being a symptom of early pregnancy, although there are plenty of descriptions of a cough being part of the diagnosis of pregnancy in older texts and in Chinese medicine, where it is considered as being part of kidney deficiency. The cough when present often leads to vomiting.

· *Heather Hill* ·

I am now eight weeks pregnant with my second child, very pleased to be pregnant and eagerly awaiting the arrival of my new child. I started being very sick and nauseous at five weeks. It starts at about midday and lasts until six although it can be longer; it is linked with extreme tiredness. I have got it much worse than last time when I was a bit tired but never sick and never nauseous.

Last time I was pregnant I was at work until 33 weeks and I do feel that it helps; you have to put the way you feel on the back burner a bit. This time I am at home and able to pamper myself a bit more, but I really had no idea that I would feel so absolutely exhausted and totally drained. The only things that help are eating little and often and getting extra sleep. If I'm able to get a couple of hours' extra sleep during the day when Callum is asleep it makes all the difference.

I'm trying to eat healthy food because I don't want to put weight on the way I did last time. I was very active until I left work and then I'd eat anything because I was so hungry. I think I took on board that thing about eating for two and I used to eat uncut bread in its naked state, or toasted with things on, muesli and oranges. I put on a stone-and-a-half in the last few weeks.

This time I'm eating fruit, oatcakes and tuna, salads etc – healthy things – but it seems to be carbohydrate that really helps. If I have an apple I often have to have a sandwich a bit later. It holds the sickness in abeyance for a while and then back it comes again.

All the symptoms are worse this time. I've got chronic indigestion and heartburn which I only got towards the end last time. It is getting a bit better although even last week was terrible. I had a particularly bad day recently when there was no getting away from it and nothing that I did made any difference. Then I really questioned being pregnant.

· Carol Ann Rogers ·

I'm nearly 12 weeks now and just feel sick all the time. The only thing that helps is eating and fizzy water. I'm probably eating a lot more than I used to, but because I'm a hairdresser I used to go for a long time without eating so I'm probably only eating about as much as I should have done before. I started feeling sick right away, before I missed a period. I just feel yucky all the time but it has not stopped me doing anything. I still exercise which probably keeps the weight off. I am alright if I eat regularly – anything will do.

A week or so later . . .

I am 13 weeks now and have stopped feeling sick. I am still running and feel much better. I've hardly put on any weight so that's not been a problem, it's just wonderful to feel semi-normal again.

· Alison Archibald ·

It started when we were sailing around the Ionian islands in Michael's 24-foot yacht. I had never sailed before apart from a few weekends away before the trip and I had been sick on those occasions – even the cat was sick – but I thought that I was getting used to it and they say that even the best sailors can take some time to get their sea legs. We set off on holiday in early June. I was immediately sick and took to my bed. The six hour journey lasted 10 hours because the boat developed a serious leak. At one point Michael, who was bailing out every 5 minutes shouted down to me that the boat was likely to sink. As I was groaning and chucking up at the time, I didn't care, and thought I might even prefer to drown. I had been car sick and this was almost the same kind of sickness. Eventually we got to the port and were able to get the boat repaired. However, the sea-sickness did not vanish when we were tied up to the pier or even on dry land and eventually we realised that it might be due to something other than motion. I travelled back to the island where we were based and did a pregnancy test, which proved positive.

By the end of August, I was so sick that we had to cut the holiday short. Michael had to sail the boat back to Paxos and I had to get back to the UK by myself. This took several days and was a nightmare while I was feeling constantly sick.

Michael was still sailing the boat back so I was on my own. Just before I left, having finally found a sympathetic holiday company, friends took me out for a meal to make me feel better and although I was often better past eight in the evening, I still found that on this occasion I needed to be sick at the side of the road. This was in a place with an 18-30 club where I'm sure they were used to seeing women being sick ten times a night but I felt absolutely awful and just wanted to be able to say, 'I'm not drunk – I'm pregnant.'

However, back home, at 17 weeks, the day after my amniocentesis which I'm sure was just coincidence, I stopped being sick: it didn't taper off, it just stopped overnight.

In fact with this pregnancy and the next, the sickness stopped at the time I first felt the baby move.

With my second pregnancy, I started to be sick within four weeks of getting pregnant. It was not as stressful as when we were sailing but this time I had Calum to cope with and it was as much as I could do to get him to nursery. I certainly could not have held down a job. I lived on breakfast cereal, I could eat breakfast and if I was lucky I could keep down a bowl for lunch. I drank gallons of orange juice and soda mixed, but I completely went off chocolate, although I am a chocoholic. The worst thing was the constancy of nausea and vomiting and the uncertainty about how long it would last or when I would be sick.

My mother's reaction was unhelpful, she had been sick when she was expecting me and my twin sister. However, she had been given a lift to work and was only sick when she saw the person who gave her the lift start up his car to pick her up. She believed that it was all in the mind, and would not occur if you got out and did things. During her second pregnancy she had 18-month-old twins to cope with and had no time to be sick, according to her. Interestingly, my twin sister, who has three girls, was sick every time until she was 17 weeks pregnant. My younger sister did not have much pregnancy sickness with either her girl or her boy, just feelings of nausea in the first few weeks – yet her childhood motion sickness was worse than ours.

With Caitlin I was sick once, by the side of the road when I was coming back from the library. In Greece I often had to find an olive tree to be sick behind.

After that I found it useful to carry airline sick bags which I got from a friend who is an air stewardess. The pattern of sickness was similar, being almost constantly sick from 4 o'clock in the afternoon until 8 o'clock at night, after which time I could keep something down. Even so, I lost at least a stone in weight and only started to gain weight once the sickness was over. It was useful to eat dry crackers but only because it is better to be sick on something rather than nothing. There is nothing worse than retching on an empty stomach.

I got used to Calum saying, 'Sicking again' and 'Did you not like that, Mummy?' and 'Spit it out into the bucket'. However, other people's regard of morning sickness as a trivial illness was illustrated by a friend whose child I cared for while she had chicken pox, but who failed to make any offer of help while I was so sick.

With Caitlin, the sickness also stopped instantly, although earlier, when I was 14 weeks pregnant, on Christmas Eve. I was still horribly sick that day and night but on Christmas Day I was able to eat like a pig, as if I had not eaten for weeks, which effectively, I hadn't. And I was never sick again.

Nothing actually made it better. I tried herb teas which didn't help; I did try the wrist bands with Caitlin but I don't know if they helped because once I had them on I daren't ever take them off in case I felt worse! The only thing that cured it was time.

· *Heather Mattock* ·

My sickness started at about five-and-a-half months; before that I was really fine. I was never actually sick, I just felt that I was going to be sick any minute. I didn't get the relief of being sick. Dizziness started at the same time but finished earlier. I did pass out a couple of times. By seven months the dizziness had gone but the nausea, which always started after midday, didn't end until just before eight months. My doctor couldn't believe it. He said it was linked with tiredness and encouraged me to get more sleep so I was going to bed at ridiculous times like 8.30. I tried it for a week but couldn't sleep – I was just lying there awake and it didn't help so I gave it up.

· *Isobel Gettings* ·

All my pregnancies were different. The first was not too bad; with the second I was actively losing weight and wanted to take Debendox *but didn't in the end. That time I felt queasy until the eighteenth week. I think it has a lot to do with how tired you are – with the boys* [her last two] *I felt sick right until 42 and 43 weeks.*

I'm not normally a sicky person; I've got a cast-iron stomach. With pregnancy, though, the very first sign, even before missing a period, was not being able to put my toothbrush in my mouth without feeling sick. Going to the dentist was terrible; he had to do the work in quick bursts.

I was highly sensitive to smells. I had to run past the butcher's and once had to dash out of the shop. I found the smell of drains particularly nauseating.

I also had that horrible taste in the mouth and I craved pickles, gherkins and cabbage – anything like that. Ginger beer helped with the nausea; Idris was the most effective.

· *Food Cravings and Aversions* ·

Food cravings and pica, which is the desire to eat things generally considered inedible, are popularly linked with pregnancy. The larger part of the research on the subject was done in the fifties when it was expected of women who were pregnant.

These days, women still experience food cravings of a very specific nature in pregnancy (see Whitehead *et al.*, 1992) but it is unusual to hear of women eating inedible things such as coal. This change in emphasis is generally ascribed to the improvement in people's diet so that they are now unlikely to be lacking a specific vitamin or mineral, although from a fascinating article based on responses to a BBC radio programme in 1956, it was clear that many of the writers had been very ashamed of their cravings at that time, and kept them quiet even from their husbands. (See Case History p. 39.)

The authors of the fifties' research, Harries and Hughes (1958), made it clear that their paper did not reflect general experience as the respondents were self-selected and there would be likely to be a bias towards the unusual. They found that the food most commonly craved was fruit (261) and then vegetables (105), usually eaten raw. Of the fruit, apples proved most popular (76), closely followed by oranges (68), other citrus fruit (24), tomatoes (31), down to plantains, pomegranates and raisins. Pickled food and cereals were next although the cereals such as macaroni, maize, rice, oatmeal and Indian corn were usually eaten raw. Interestingly, of the 991 cases, 17 craved alcohol as well as milk and milk products.

The more bizarre food cravings included coffee grounds (5), fat (3), tea leaves (2), aspirin, coconut milk, custard powder, dog biscuits, health salts, jelly and stomach powder.

Other unusual substances craved include coal, the most popular (35), soap (17), disinfectant (15), toothpaste (14), mothballs (10), petrol, metal polish, tar, paraffin, wood, soil, chalk, charcoal, cinders and others – all the above were desired by at least 4 women.

The aversions, of which there were 193, listed things that the mothers normally enjoyed but disliked during pregnancy. Tea topped the list (78), followed by tobacco, smoking, coffee (22) and marmalade (8). Chocolates, eggs and sweet food followed while beer, the only alcohol mentioned, was only disliked by 4 (although perhaps fewer women would normally drink regularly at that time).

Most cravings were experienced in the first four months, usually fairly early on. It was clear that the cravings were intense and specific. Women often felt able to joke about them after the birth but found them so overpowering at the time that they had to indulge them even if they could not afford them or were tempted to steal to satisfy their longings.

At about the same time Posner *et al.* (1957) analysed cravings and pica by taking 600 consecutive women in Harlem and questioning them about their specific desires. All were in the third trimester of pregnancy: 394 admitted cravings, 196 denied it and 10 admitted pica.

Top of the cravings list was Argo starch, a brand of corn flour (106), then sweets, particularly chocolate nut bars (68). Next were fruits and juices, ice, Pepsi Cola, some pickles, meats and chicken (13), carbonated sodas (12), down to Vick's cough drops (12). One of the women craving baking soda, who hardly baked normally, was consuming as much as 12 oz per week. Of those with pica, eight ate red clay, one ate white clay and one ate pencil erasers. Coral Jepson, a midwife working for ARHTAG, a health education programme, described African women in the early stages of pregnancy picking up handfuls of red soil and eating them freely.

Posner *et al.* found that women with run-of-the-mill cravings felt free to admit them to their families whereas the most unusual ones were kept secret. The women felt unable to resist them even when they feared they might harm themselves or their baby. No evidence of their having been harmful was discovered. It may be that in these more health-conscious times, when even a drop of alcohol is advised against by some health professionals, the potentially damaging or bizarre-sounding pica has gone underground.

More recently, Hook (1978) interviewed 250 women in New York State about their cravings and aversions. Most desired was ice cream (46), chocolate (39), citrus fruit and juices (39) and sweets. Only six women wanted salty foods. Hook charts the desired food against food women were averse to, which is of interest because something as apparently nutritious as poultry was disliked by 42 women but wanted by 14. He speculates that as women 'go off' things that are known to be toxic to the fetus, such as smoking and alcohol, these alterations in taste perception may have a protective function, and certainly more of his sample gave up alcohol because it was unpleasant to taste rather than for reasons of concern for their health or that of their baby. He emphasises that it should not be assumed that foods to which women develop aversion are toxic until direct evidence is available (although there seems nothing to be gained by forcing yourself to eat something that you currently dislike). It may be that cravings and aversion are subtly tuned to each pregnancy and should be obeyed unless common sense suggests they may be injurious.

On the other hand it may be due to similar factors to those which cause nausea and vomiting. Whitehead *et al.* (1992), in their study of a thousand women interviewed while still pregnant, found that women who developed food cravings were more likely to develop nausea. They did not encounter a single case of pica. Davies & Stewart (1987) state that zinc deficiency is associated with impairment of taste and smell.

Whether cravings and aversions are messages about the intrinsic needs of you and your baby, warnings about what might be harmful, or merely a further disturbance of your system caused by being pregnant is not clear. However, if obeying them makes you feel better, it seems to make sense to do it. Liliana Stark (p. 42) found it helpful to pinch or bite a spot between her index finger and thumb – or get someone else to do it for her. Later she discovered that this covers the spot reflexologists regard as relating to the stomach.

· *Lisa Kinsella* ·

I did try and eat coal – it wasn't for the taste but the texture. I really wanted to crunch it and said to my husband once in the middle of the night, that I had got to do it. But it was disappointing because we had the wrong kind, it was preformed like 50 pence pieces, not like the proper stuff. I wanted something like cinders – after that my friend used to offer me the freedom of her coal bunker.

It wasn't the only thing I craved: I also chewed ice cubes all the way through. I bought bags and bags of those kilo bags of ice from Sainsbury's, and my mum had to put trays of ice ready for me when I went round to see her.

I went mad trying to buy those crumbly mints that are a bit like Edinburgh rock but I couldn't find them anywhere. I did once eat half a stick of chalk, and I would chew paracetamol tablets and spit them out when they were chewed. I took Gaviscon tablets too, just for the pleasure of crunching them. It only happened with the girls though, I didn't get it with Kieran.

· *Emotional Aspects* ·

The physical effects of pregnancy sickness can be overwhelming but it can also have all sorts of emotional or social ramifications. Becoming or feeling ill, for what may seem a very long time, can put you into a very different role to that which you adopt normally and you may wonder whether pregnancy is worth it if it has such dire consequences.

Firstly, it is very unusual for anyone to be consistently ill without the illness being serious and recognised as such. In situations where you are labelled as being really ill recommendations would be made about rest, probably in bed; you would be given time off work with a sick note and your family and friends would accept that some of your responsibilities would have to be shouldered by them.

With pregnancy sickness, though you may feel dreadfully ill, the whole thing is on a different footing. It may be that you do not want to tell people yet, either because it may have a bearing on your employment, or because you want to be as sure as possible that you will not miscarry before telling the world (though women who do miscarry before they have announced their pregnancy sometimes regret not having told people). In that situation, no one else can be blamed for not taking your sickness seriously. However, it is clear from the stories that women tell that they may not be treated as properly ill even if they do declare their problem.

Medical staff may be happy to come out with such palliatives as '*emesis gravidarum* (normal pregnancy sickness) is usually well-tolerated by patients following explanation and reassurance that it is likely to be short-lived and that it is a good indicator of fetal outcome (healthy baby)': or this, from a handout from the American Academy of Family Physicians – 'If these steps (dry cracker routine) don't give you relief from morning sickness your doctor may have other ideas. Keep in mind that your symptoms should go away soon and that morning sickness doesn't mean your baby is sick.'

It can be hard for other people to imagine unrelenting sickness and they will want or prefer you to be happy about the forthcoming baby. As Michael says (p. 107) you are deemed to have brought it on yourself which is not the case with illness, which may be seen as an act of God and unavoidable.

Pregnancy does have an effect on your emotional state: the Avon study showed that women often found themselves being more irritable. It is less easy to tolerate other people's demands when you feel as if you are in a permanent state of premenstrual tension and sick to boot. It can be particularly irritating to have people attributing sickness to psychological factors.

Although the school of thought which attributes symptoms to the hysterical, neurotic nature of the mother is in decline it evidently still holds some sway. Most sufferers would agree that there is a slight psychological component; many felt better at work, when they were distracted or when in hospital with all their other responsibilities off their shoulders. Nearly everyone managed to contain their sickness until they could reach something to be sick into.

Some people were actually glad to be suffering from pregnancy sickness, particularly if they had miscarried before and not felt as sick in those pregnancies. It can be a positive sign in this instance, although it is still possible to miscarry after having awful pregnancy sickness as some of the mothers in the stories show, and many women have no symptoms and go happily to full term. However, there is a lower rate of miscarriage among those who have severe pregnancy sickness. One woman said 'I was absolutely delighted to be so sick because after a period of infertility and two miscarriages, it meant that it looked as if I was really going to have a baby.'

· *Nic Rauh* ·

I was amazed when I went to my antenatal classes to find that no one had had it as badly as me. I used to have two bad days and then a day off and then another couple of bad days and so on. I went to my doctor and told her about it and she just suggested dry biscuits by the bed. I had been sick three times while I waited to see her – all she said was 'you poor woman' – I wanted someone to hug me. There was no way that I could have worked while I still had it. To begin with I was working front of house at the National – I told the manager that I was pregnant and was sick at the same time. They were very sympathetic.

I remember sitting beside the pool in Spain and really giving up for a couple of hours. I just couldn't see how I was going to be a mum if I felt so dreadful. It was worse than any flu. I recall going to tell my friend that I was pregnant, on a beautiful spring day but I know I looked dreadful, dressed like a bag lady. On another occasion we went to the cinema after eating a huge roast. I felt a bit odd and had a fizzy drink and then was taken completely by surprise by the vomiting. I was sick seven times in an hour; it was just like petrol at the end, it was so violent.

I love food and it was as if my body was reacting against me, the little embryo was like an alien. I was astonished to learn that in some cultures, such as that in Papua New Guinea, they just don't get pregnancy sickness. Mine was textbook though, by fifteen weeks it had gone. In the second trimester I was superwoman! I started rehearsals just as it waned.

· *Liliana Stark* ·

I have had five pregnancies and three abortions and it got worse with each one. With the first pregnancy my mother realised that I was pregnant before I did because I was being sick all the time (my mother did not suffer from pregnancy sickness). I was sick right until I had the abortion and it didn't stop for a couple of days afterwards, but the relief was considerable. The second time I had an abortion really early. I was very sick when I took the contraceptive pill.

Thirteen-and-a-half years ago I had Kylie. It was a long time since the first pregnancy and although I was sick straightaway, I thought it was a bug: this was in Israel. Eventually I was admitted to hospital and was in for three months. I was bleeding a lot too, the pressure of being sick constantly made me bleed. They put me on Maxolon tablets which they said were the safest, but I couldn't keep them down so I had to have it by injection and be drip-fed. The Maxolon did numb my stomach and stop me actually being sick. After three months it started to ease off although I continued to be sick right up to the birth and a bit after.

The next pregnancy was horrendous. I knew I was pregnant twenty-four hours after I conceived – the pregnancy wasn't planned. The nausea was very aggressive, it started the moment I opened my eyes and I would vomit immediately. I went to my doctor who was convinced that it couldn't be due to pregnancy so soon and did blood tests for infection. I was hospitalised a week after that because I had become so dehydrated. I couldn't even swallow my saliva, even the thought made me heave and I had to spit it out continually.

I had an ultrasound: the baby was very tiny, the size of a thumb-nail. I had to be put on a drip. The doctors were very unsympathetic: they said that I wanted an abortion and was trying to jump the queue. When I said that this wasn't so and that although it was unplanned I was happy to have the baby, they said that I wanted it too much. My husband said that if they were so sure that it was caused by mental problems they should get a psychiatrist to see me.

I felt so ill that I just wanted to die. There was a South African doctor on the ward who was very opposed to abortion and he wanted to drag it out to three months: he was really unhelpful. Eventually I left and had a private abortion in order to stop feeling so ill.

We had tried all sorts of things to make it better and spent a lot of money on hypnotherapy which didn't work at all, only made it worse. In fact I used to come home and turn the washing machine on while I was vomiting so that Paul couldn't hear me throwing up £30.

After three months I found that I couldn't come to terms with having had an abortion so the next pregnancy was planned. If possible it was ten times worse. The same cycle repeated itself, even the slightest movement caused nausea so that I was afraid even to move in case I vomited. It was so bad that I was vomiting blood. I was in hospital for three months again and Kylie had to go to a childminder.

I was on a drip at Ealing hospital for a few weeks to start with. They couldn't work out what was wrong; they thought that it might be twins or that my blood might be incompatible with my husband's (although it had happened with the pregnancies that weren't his), or that it was due to a mental disorder.

People's attitudes were awful in England: Mediterranean people were more sympathetic. Here doctors won't believe you and then when they have the evidence they treat pregnancy sickness as a mental problem.

I lost a lot of weight (33lb). Eventually I was transferred to Chelsea hospital where they did more scans and tests. I was still on a drip and they were getting worried that it would affect the health of the baby. Just as I was approaching three months they moved me to Guy's where they were going to put me in a special unit for accident victims who were fed through the neck. They fed me protein intravenously at Guy's. They kept trying to feed me normally but I couldn't keep anything down. I didn't eat anything properly for weeks. As I reached three months it got a little bit better but it still continued until after the birth.

I remember feeling hungry and miserable and dreaming of Chinese food. I got so wretched that I wanted to jump out of the window. I slept a lot.

There were considerable side-effects besides losing all that weight: my teeth fell out – I've got thirteen crowns now; my hair fell out and my skin was very dry. It affected my eyesight and memory and I've got holes in my arms where the drips went in.

The babies were born early: two weeks early by my dates and six and four weeks early by theirs. I wasn't surprised, all the pressure of being sick seemed as though it must push them out. They weren't small: Kylie was 6lb 1oz and Ben was 6lb 3oz but their baby teeth were damaged.

I read up a lot about it and so tried crushed ice, which was recommended. It did help with the heartburn a bit but not with the sickness. Sweeties and chewing gum helped me to swallow saliva, it was the only way that I could swallow. I ate hundreds of sweeties. My mother-in-law cooked me things that were hard to vomit like liver, and rice but I was still sick.

I found my sense of smell became very acute. I could smell things like a match which had been struck in the park five minutes before and cigarettes were fatal, I couldn't go near anyone smoking. I wasn't any fun to be near either!

The only cure for me was orange juice – just like the old Jewish joke where a woman goes to her doctor and says, 'I don't want to have any more children' and he says, 'Try orange juice.' Just as she is leaving she says, 'Before or after?' and he says, 'Instead'!

Chapter Four

HYPEREMESIS GRAVIDARUM

Hyperemesis gravidarum is the name for severe vomiting in pregnancy. It is thought to affect 5–10 women in a thousand, and is defined as persistent vomiting that interferes with nutrition, fluid and electrolyte balance. It is potentially very serious as uncontrolled vomiting can be fatal, and it is only since the technique of giving intravenous fluids has been perfected that women have stopped dying as a consequence of having the condition.

In practice, *hyperemesis gravidarum* is diagnosed when a mother's condition is sufficiently serious to warrant admission to hospital and that seems partly dependent on the woman and her doctor. If you have lost more than 5% of your pre-pregnancy weight through vomiting you can be described as having *hyperemesis gravidarum* (see p. 21 for other signs and symptoms). You may be vomiting 3–4 times a day or much more often, definitions vary, but you will have been being sick for at least several days, will be weak, tired and unable to work. You may look grey and emaciated and have a headache caused by dehydration.

Women often improve a little, simply by being in hospital, resting, with their other responsibilities taken off their shoulders. A series of tests are done for haemoglobin, full blood count, urea, sugar, liver function, electrolyte balance, and a urine test for ketones.

Treatment is by putting up a saline drip, possibly containing glucose, drugs to stop the vomiting, and possibly vitamins. Correcting nutritional deficiencies by adding multivitamins has been shown to improve symptoms within 24 hours (van Stuijvenberg, 1995).

The likely course of events should you need to be admitted is that your attacks of vomiting will gradually cease over several days and you will then be offered a liquid diet. If you are able to retain this you will be offered a light semi-liquid diet. By the time you can tolerate eating and are starting to gain weight you will be able to leave. In most cases women continue to improve but some have to be readmitted as they relapse when back at home. Some researchers consider weight gain to be the best indicator of whether you are likely to continue to get better or relapse.

It is important to be sure that your vomiting is due to pregnancy alone, so while in hospital you should be offered ultrasound to check that you have not got a molar pregnancy, or to see if there is more than one baby. (Other possible causes of symptoms are mentioned on p. 22.)

Vomiting of such severity is likely to cause you anxiety, both on your own behalf and for the safety of your baby. The following chapter discusses these issues.

· *Denise Payne* ·

My first pregnancy with Louis was no real problem. I did have nausea in the morning; I used to get that awful rolling feeling until I'd had something like cereal to eat. I found if I neglected to eat regularly, I would feel light-headed, not up to par.

It started at about six weeks and lasted until 12 weeks, but was nothing out of the ordinary.

I was ill at around 30 weeks. I got a stomach bug and couldn't stop myself being sick so I was admitted to hospital and put on a drip for a couple of days. They said it would just have to work its way out of my system, and that's what happened.

With my second pregnancy I felt sick as soon as it was possible to – about the time I missed a period. I have no clear memory of actually vomiting before 14–15 weeks. One Friday morning, just before lunch, I had to collect Louis from nursery and I just sat down and thought I've got to rest. My mind had almost disengaged when I looked at the clock and thought I must get Louis. I stood up and thought I had wet myself. I went hurtling to the loo genuinely thinking I was just wet and pulled down my pants to find blood everywhere. I was shocked and frightened but phoned a friend who said ring the doctor at once. I saved everything. The doctor came, listened with her stethoscope, prodded my tummy and said, 'Yes, I think you've lost the baby. The best thing to do is move around as much as possible so it will go of its own accord.' I did do that, but by Monday I felt so ill I couldn't move and I was still feeling very sick.

We went to the surgery where she did an ultrasound and said, 'Yes, you've definitely lost the baby'. Matthew said to her that I was so ill I needed to be seen by someone and it was arranged that I went to hospital that afternoon. There I was examined by a consultant obstetrician who thought that I had lost the baby but also had a cyst on one of my ovaries. I was still feeling awful and it was arranged that I should go to theatre that afternoon for a D & C and laparoscopy, just to make sure of the cyst.

I had had my pre-med and went down to the ante-room for the operation. While I was there the anaesthetist, who was looking through my notes, asked me which side the cyst was. I said that I didn't know. He said, 'I'll just run the ultrasound over your tummy to make sure.' As he did that he went very quiet and then looked at my notes again. Then he said, 'How many weeks pregnant are you?' and I told him 14–15 weeks. Then he said, 'Tell me again what you're in here for' and I told him it was for incomplete abortion and cyst on my ovary. He said, 'Well, this cyst looks as if it's got arms and legs and is doing cartwheels' and he turned the screen towards me and there was Saskia. There was a big black circle as well and he said that I had probably been carrying non-identical twins. The problem was that the cervix was open and if the placenta decided to come away all at once then the force could bring the other one with it. He suggested I went home and had complete rest so that it would drip away and as the live twin grew it would push everything else out of the way.

I went back to the ward where the consultant said, 'I can't guarantee that you will go full term. It's your decision – you can have a termination and start again or go with it and what will be, will be.'

I said to Matthew, 'It's here, I don't want to end it. If it does go it will be an experience and we will have to accommodate our lives around it.'

However from that time on, even while I was still at the hospital, I was continually sick. I was sick morning, noon and night – I'd even wake at three in the morning to be sick. The sickness was more violent than large in volume.

I used to spend my day sleeping. Matthew would come home and cook something like boiled fish and potatoes or vegetables. Twenty minutes later it was back again. It was a really upsetting time. I had a bulging tummy but was losing blood all the time. I felt the sickness meant that I was not helping the baby. My midwife explained that in fact the baby would take what it wanted from me and that it was myself that I would have to look after.

I tried to eat but all I could manage was Complan, *digestive biscuits and rich tea biscuits, ginger beer and tonic water. A homeopath suggested tea made from ginger root which I tried but it was really more than I could cope with. It seemed particularly strong. I don't normally touch ginger biscuits or cake but the ginger didn't taste the same in ginger beer, which did help. The tonic water helped because of the fizz. Nothing appealed to me – if I could have had food in tablet form, I would have done. I did find* Floradix *(herbal iron preparation) useful. If I took ordinary iron it made me feel a bit sick and made me constipated and they didn't want me to strain because of the risk of losing the baby.*

I had an awful taste in my mouth and my gums bled a lot everytime I cleaned my teeth. In fact I had to have a lot of dental work done afterwards because my gums were so tender and had receded. My dentist suspected I had bulimia and I had to explain what had caused the vomiting.

The sickness meant that I always had to have a bucket at the side of the bed. I'd wake up in the middle of the night and lie completely still so as not to be sick. I hate being sick: they can do anything else to me, inject me – anything, but I can't bear being sick. I'd grab Matthew's hand and say, 'I'm going to be sick again.'

Louis found it very upsetting as, of course, family life wasn't brilliant. He was upset when I was sick and he would try to get into bed with me and I had to say, 'No' because I was frightened of being kicked in the stomach.

At 28–30 weeks it did stop. It gradually tailed off over 10 days and although I occasionally got that woozy feeling, I was never sick again.

I was ill for so long, although people kept telling me that it would be over soon, when I started to show, or when I got to a certain number of weeks, but none of it was true.

Saskia was born exactly a month early. She was due on 8th April and arrived on 8th March, a healthy 6lb 7oz. My midwife suggested that the sickness might have been because she was a girl or because it had been twins, but we'll never know.

· *Kirsten Johnson* ·
(see also Mark Elliott, p.106)

I was about 7–8 weeks pregnant for the first time when I had a big bleed. I was taken into hospital ending up in the Ear, Nose and Throat ward because there was no other bed available, and kept in overnight. The following morning I started to be sick. I had been a bit nauseous before but I was so sick that they kept me in for two days and put me on a drip. After two days I went home but I was still being sick, as much as a dozen times a day.

This happened just as I took over temporarily from my boss who was on a long holiday. I had only done the job for a few days when I was admitted and then I didn't go back for six weeks. We were short-staffed anyway, and I probably missed an opportunity, although they were very good about the amount of time I was off sick.

All I could do was lie down at home. I couldn't even keep sips of water down, let alone the tablets I was given. I was virtually bedridden for six weeks being continually sick, feeling particularly alone and useless. I didn't know many people because we had recently moved into the area, and although the doctors were sympathetic, there was no real understanding or support.

Nothing really helped. I had a horrible taste in my mouth right the way through pregnancy. At the start, when I was beginning to be nauseous, I wanted to eat fruit sweets to get a fresh fruity taste in my mouth. I even ate Opal Fruits although I am a vegetarian and never normally eat gelatine.

I went off mint and ginger although both are recommended for sickness. I had to get a children's toothpaste flavoured with blackcurrant instead of the usual mint one. Cleaning my teeth was difficult. I wanted to because of being sick so much, but it could make me sick. I think it's because you hold your breath to clean your teeth and can't swallow.

I also found that I couldn't go into the kitchen or open the fridge door.

I could even be nauseated by the smell of the spices in the cupboard if Mark opened it while I was in the bedroom. If I had a good day and could tolerate some food it had to be incredibly bland, like jacket potato and cottage cheese, or plain pasta and broccoli. I went off real coffee which I usually enjoy, but fortunately none of these aversions lasted past the birth.

Mark was brilliant – he even used to rub my back while I was throwing up – I couldn't do that for him. But it was very difficult as I had become pregnant the week he started a new job in Northamptonshire. Normally he would spend one night a week there but he used to come back every night and sort the house out, and he kept in contact with my office. It was a big strain. My mother was good too; she came for a week's holiday and stayed for three weeks to look after me. She had been sick right through two pregnancies although she was not as bad as I was.

I was admitted for rehydration three times altogether. Things would gradually get worse over 2–3 days and we'd call the doctor who had me admitted. They did try tablets and suppositories. I couldn't keep the tablets down and even the suppositories seemed to make no difference at all. Everyone kept saying, 'You're very unlucky but it will stop at three months' and then, 'Well, with some unfortunate people it goes on to four months' and they kept pushing the time barriers back. Finally they said, 'At least you know it will be over by February.'

The drip put me off having an epidural in labour. It was horrible having the needle in. It made it hard to move and sleeping was difficult because I normally sleep with my hand beneath me. One night a nurse twisted the tubing of the drip to encourage the fluid to move an air bubble and this sent an excruciating pain down my arm. I could get about with the drip as it was on wheels, but I felt so weak that I didn't want to move.

The second time I was admitted was during a really hot spell. I was in the post-operative gynaecology ward with women who had had hysterectomies and terminations. They were all wondering why I was there, and as it was so hot and I felt sick I had the only fan in the room, which I felt led to some resentment.

The last time I was there I was in the maternity unit with two other women suffering from the same thing. We had someone in with us who was full-term and healthy and about to be induced, which was quite strange. It was only after this last visit that I seem to remember being told that if I was very sick again I should just come straight to the Maternity Unit and bypass Casualty.

I only remember being weighed once at the first visit to the antenatal clinic, but I guess I lost at least a stone or more. I felt very thin and didn't put much weight on at all; I was back into my ordinary clothes a week after the birth.

Whenever I got up I felt very weak and used to throw up in the car on the way to the hospital. I'd keep plastic bags in the car. The worst time was when I was admitted to Casualty and had to lie there being sick. I was sick twice when they put me in the milk float thing to transfer me to the ward. Obviously, I was reluctant to go out for fear of being sick in public. I had felt very sick travelling to Aberdeen when I was five months pregnant – as soon as I got off the plane on our return I was horrifically sick and had to be taken off in a wheelchair. It was so embarrassing.

The whole thing took away nine months out of my life; I only felt reasonable for one week. I was off work for two months: after the first sick note ran out, I went back but only managed a day, and had to stay off for the rest of the week.

By the end I was still nauseous, I was anaemic, I had terrible heartburn and I had back problems due to ligament pains which were sorted out by a chiropractor.

I had a 20-hour drug-free labour – it wasn't fun but I'd rather do it 10 times over again than go through that pregnancy. The moment Flora was born the feeling of sickness went. I had tea and toast and I couldn't believe that the taste in my mouth had gone and I didn't feel sick. She weighed 8lb 7oz so didn't suffer from being low birthweight. However, she does have a bowel problem and I worry that the drugs I took could have caused it, or that the excessive vomiting deprived her of something in the womb.

The long-term effect is on my hair which has lost its curl – although it might be returning now Flora is 18 months old – and on the way I feel about being pregnant. I'd love to have another baby. I don't want to leave it too long but I'm terrified of being pregnant. I have always hated being sick and could never understand people making themselves sick deliberately for whatever reason. I would have liked some follow-up or referral so that I had some idea of what the chances were of it happening again, or if there's anything that could be done to prevent it.

People don't understand: they think I'm exaggerating, or say, 'You were a bit sick when you were pregnant, weren't you?' Then they look at Flora and say, 'Well, she's worth it, isn't she?' and I wonder.

I resent people who have a trouble-free pregnancy and can continue their lives as normal throughout. I would have loved to have enjoyed carrying Flora.

· *Laura Scowsill* ·

Over the last eight years I have had four pregnancies, one of which I miscarried at nine weeks. With each pregnancy I suffered severe nausea and vomiting and became hospitalised due to dehydration.

To make matters worse I was suffering from a post-viral syndrome (ME, or Chronic Fatigue Syndrome). I first became ill in 1988, after I had been married for two months. I spent the days lying down. My doctor gave me medication for the nausea. This helped a little, but I was still very weak, and could only walk a little way, from one piece of furniture to another. I had not intended to become pregnant, and it is quite amazing that I was able to conceive.

Due to the pregnancy, I had to come off the medication. I had to cope with the nausea from the ME, and then the pregnancy nausea, which also involved severe vomiting. The pregnancy was so important to me that I was prepared to suffer the pain that the ME caused.

At around six months the vomiting stopped and the pain from the nausea decreased. I went to term and delivered a healthy baby boy.

The second pregnancy was once again unplanned, starting when my first baby, William, was only seven months. I no longer had the painful nausea from the ME, only extreme tiredness, coupled with an impaired immune system. I caught every cold and had numerous bouts of gastro-enteritis, urine infections and so on. But once again the pregnancy nausea started at six weeks, and I was vomiting severely until 14 weeks. I ended up in hospital at twelve weeks being rehydrated. At forty weeks I delivered another healthy baby boy.

Six years passed and I began to make good progress as far as the ME was concerned. We then decided to have another baby, hopefully this time I would sail through the pregnancy as I was so much stronger. Unfortunately this pregnancy was not to be and I miscarried. I never suffered any nausea during the six to nine weeks that I was pregnant!

We tried again and this time it worked: I was pregnant! But once again I got to six weeks and the nausea reared its ugly head. I then went through three months of severe vomiting coupled with nausea, only to be hospitalised once again to be rehydrated.

I cannot understand how anyone with real pregnancy sickness can carry on going to work, shopping and cooking, as I could not even stand up without vomiting. Drinking water was the worst, as it tasted so acidic, I could not even swallow it without vomiting. It used to burn as it went down into my stomach. I lived on the blandest food available, but that nearly always came back, except sometimes, if I lay really still for about two hours it would stay down if I was lucky. The usual smells like perfume and cooking were horrendous.

In every pregnancy, I had to have my parents live with us, in order to take care of the children. It was a complete disruption to our lives. I was helpless, and I felt so frustrated lying on my bed, unable to care for my family. The effect it had on my husband and children, not to mention my parents who had to drop everything and care for us, was devastating.

All the time I was unable to care for my family, I felt so angry that there was nothing available to help me through this period, and that the attitude from the medical staff was that the nausea was perfectly healthy and that you just had to get on with it and wait for it to subside.

Chapter Five

WHAT IS THE EFFECT ON MOTHER AND BABY?

Surprisingly little has been written about long-term effects on mothers who have had *hyperemesis gravidarum*, although the women who describe it in this book mention problems with teeth and hair which have lasted past the birth.

During the pregnancy, apart from feeling ghastly, there seem to be two conditions that can be caused by frequent vomiting: vaginal bleeding and premature contractions. It is also possible, although very unusual, for the extreme pressure of constant vomiting to rupture the oesophagus.

Research has found that women with bleeding and premature contractions have gone on to have pregnancies with no more complications and their babies were no worse off than those in the control group (Bashiri *et al.*, 1995). Much more work has been done on the effects that *hyperemesis gravidarum* has on the baby, and whether drugs given to counteract it give rise to any abnormalities. As is consistent with other research into pregnancy sickness, results are conflicting, but the majority of babies did not appear to suffer from their mothers' illness.

On the positive side, the studies showed that miscarriage and still-birth rates were lower in women with *hyperemesis gravidarum*. There also is a smaller chance of having an ectopic pregnancy, although this may only mean that you do not get severe nausea and vomiting if your pregnancy is ectopic (see Christine Asbury's story p. 111). A study of 3000 women by Kallen (1987) in Sweden showed that such babies were born slightly earlier than average but that their risk of dying around the time of birth was no greater than that of babies whose mothers did not have pregnancy sickness. Two studies (Brandes, 1967; Klebanoff *et al.*, 1985) found that babies of *hyperemesis gravidarum* mothers were larger than average and that 18% (as opposed to 5.3%) of these babies were heavier than 4000gm (8lb 13oz).

Another study separated 64 women into groups depending on weight loss: one group that lost more than 5% of their pre-pregnancy weight and another that lost less (Gross *et al.* 1989). Babies of the severe loss group were likely to be lighter that those in the other group, some being considered growth-retarded. Three of the babies in the severe group had minor abnormalities such as webbed toes, an extra finger and skin tags. The women had been treated with *Stemetil*, *Phenergan*, doxylamine and pyridoxine.

Pettitti (1986) also found that babies of women who had *hyperemesis gravidarum* all the way through pregnancy were more likely to have abnormalities and be growth-retarded. On the other hand, Klebanoff and Mills (1986) found no association between teratogenicity (fetal abnormalities caused by adverse factors in early pregnancy) and vomiting. They raised the question of whether it is better to treat *hyperemesis gravidarum* with drugs, when there is a small risk of causing abnormality, rather than allowing the vomiting to continue, and letting the baby suffer from poor nutrition. They did not find any abnormalities caused by the medication although they recognised the need for a larger study.

Psychological issues, such as how the mother feels about the baby and future pregnancies, do not seem to have been covered, although these are of considerable importance to mothers themselves (see Chapter Twelve, *Your next pregnancy*, p. 114).

Chapter Six

WHAT CAUSES MORNING SICKNESS?

Researchers have been speculating on the cause of nausea and vomiting in pregnancy for more than 4000 years, since it was described on a papyrus. I am indebted to Beverley O'Brien for her work on the analysis of the historical attributes of morning sickness (O'Brien & Newton, 1991). Surprisingly, beyond the fact that it is caused by being pregnant, people are still not certain exactly why women get it, why some get it worse than others and why a few get it so severely as to require treatment in hospital without which it could be fatal.

It may seem obvious that it is caused by changing hormone levels, and there is a relationship there, but it is not necessarily proven to be cause and effect. Aristotle was the first person we know to have recorded that most pregnant women suffered nausea, headaches, feelings of heaviness in all parts of the body, sensations of darkness before the eyes, superfluous humours (swellings), rapid mood changes and longings. He appreciated that symptoms could start as soon as 10 days after a missed period and he thought symptoms were at their worst when the fetus's hair was beginning to grow. He considered that menses or periods became re-routed towards the breast to become milk. He said that a pregnant woman would be pale and experience more symptoms if the baby she was expecting was a girl (see Ross, 1988).

Soranus of Ephesus (98–138 AD) described a condition he called pica (which nowadays is a word used to describe food craving in pregnancy, particularly for things generally considered inedible) (see Temkin, 1956). He described it as deriving from an upset, fluid-filled stomach, beginning around the fortieth day and lasting for four months. All women with it were affected by a loss of appetite for certain foods, a desire for unlikely foods, such as charcoal, excessive salivation, acid eruction (burps), slowness of digestion, rapid decomposition of food, vomiting at intervals or after each meal, dizziness, pallor, headache, constipation and slight fever. Some also had signs of jaundice.

His remarkably accurate picture was based on a culture of observation, and he did not put forward a theory for the cause but regarded it as normal but among 'many inconveniences which beset the woman who is heavily burdened and suffers from pica'.

In 1665 Dr Chamberlain writing in *Dr. Chamberlain's Midwifes Practice: or a Guide for Women in that High Concern of Conception, Breeding and Nursing Children* (published evocatively as: 'London: printed for Thomas Rookls at the Lamb and Inkbottle, at the left end of St. Pauls, London') mentions the 'loathing of meat' by the pregnant woman. Symptoms normally occurred in the morning after the body was 'a little stirred'. The cause was thought to be due to bad diet, crude humours (bodily fluids) and fomentine (stimulated) blood.

Burton (1751) recognised that pregnancy also caused faintness, pains in the stomach and groin and breasts, shortness of breath and a cough which occurred early in pregnancy and abated around the third month. He took a sympathetic view of the menstrual cycle, generally stating that 'when we see the disorders brought frequently on women at the period when the menses are about to flow and what mischiefs almost constantly attend their obstruction, we need not be surprised at the faintings, reaching to vomit, etc that so often attack women in their first months of pregnancy.'

He thought that undigested food in the stomach led to irritation; excessive and 'acrimonious' food caused vomiting in pregnancy but most vomiting in pregnancy was due to compressed nerves, and that later vomiting was caused by the distended uterus and compression of the fetal head which interrupted peristalsis and was unlikely to stop before delivery.

Montgomery (1837) considered vomiting to be caused by reflex irritation from the gravid womb and 'diseased conditions of the sexual system' but Curtis (1837) thought that it was caused by irritation of the stomach which could result in vomiting and purging (diarrhoea) in the early and middle months. It could be caused by bad food, cold phlegm, constipation and uterine irritability.

Tanner (1868) observed that symptoms could start as early as 3–4 days after conception but that most started around the fourth week. Symptoms were most distressing in the early part of the day, lasting from a few minutes to a few hours. He noticed that women often wanted to eat as soon as they had vomited and recommended that they stay in bed for a short time after breakfast. He considered it due to 'sympathetic gastric irritability'.

As time went by pregnancy sickness was ascribed to more bizarre causes, and increasingly was thought to be caused by the sufferers' own psychological make-up. Coperman (1875) declared 'obstinate' nausea and vomiting to be due to increased rigidity of the cervix and claimed it could be helped by dilating the cervix with the finger.

Atkinson (1882) took a more kindly view of it, considering it due to sympathetic disturbances of the stomach in early pregnancy and direct pressure on the stomach later on. He recommended stimulants such as brandy, and care in choosing digestible foods. Belladonna and morphine were prescribed, applied rectally or to the cervix if they could not be kept down orally. He describes a colleague applying a gentle electric current from the epigastrum to the spine.

He aimed to 'make pregnancy so comfortable that the ordinary objection to this condition on the part of the woman may be greatly lessened'.

In contrast to his encouraging approach, Kaltenbach (1891) considered that women who suffered from the severest form of pregnancy sickness, *hyperemesis gravidarum*, were undergoing, or expressing unconsciously and symbolically, an abhorrence of impregnation, and loathing of the husband and the expected child. He must have considered it a powerful emotion as this was his considered opinion given after examining their bodies at post-mortem.

By 1918 Duncan and Harding were starting to be concerned about mild nausea and vomiting because it was recognised that it could lead to severe or, as it was then known, 'pernicious' vomiting, with serious or fatal consequences. They initiated high carbohydrate diets with administration of glucose or lactose.

By 1920 Titus was giving high carbohydrate diet and glucose in sodium bicarbonate apparently effectively (Titus & Givens, 1920).

In 1932 there was a *BiSoDol* symposium on the subject when many papers were presented. The most unusual theories included one in which it was claimed that the toxin (nausea and vomiting was considered to be a toxaemia of pregnancy) was derived from the male element in the fertilised ovum, and other theories included sickness being due to women demonstrating the pregnancy or showing resentment to their spouses for what they must suffer (BiSoDol, 1932).

The most clear-cut and callous extrapolation of blaming the pregnant woman came from Atlee in 1934 whose 'treatment' resulted in 'curing' 29 women, but also in therapeutic abortion for two and the death of two others in his treatment. The women who were diagnosed as having pernicious vomiting were separated from their families, largely by being admitted to hospital. They were forbidden basins in which to be sick and were made to vomit on to their beds, which he instructed were not to be cleaned up for some time afterwards.

They were informed that an abortion must not be performed under any circumstances and they were given ordinary food at mealtimes. Glucose injections were given if women were very dehydrated. Fortunately it did not become the treatment of choice.

Robertson (1946) found that women were better off if they did not speak English or adopt the culture of English speakers. McCammon (1951) found a lower incidence among American Indians with a staple diet of maize and assumed language and culture was the cause. Acquiring English language and culture would cause pregnancy sickness. Psychiatric examination of women with *hyperemesis gravidarum* (Harvey & Sherfey, 1954) concluded that sufferers were remarkably immature and frigid, and were increasingly anxious and tense in pregnancy.

A study by Coppen & Brist (1959) showed that women who experienced vomiting in pregnancy were likely to be slightly more male in their body measurements and in a later study (1963) found that vomiting women were ambivalent in their attitude to their babies. Hardly surprising if they were, but this was not discovered to be the case when the research was reassessed.

Fairweather (1965, 1968, 1978), who has examined the subject in minute detail, seems to be sympathetic to sufferers, although he considers that many of them are women of below average intelligence.

By 1971 it was beginning to be recognised that the support of the partner is helpful (Semmens, 1971) and in 1978 Wolkind and Zajicek observed that women with prolonged nausea appear to be receiving less support from their husbands or parents. Theories of psychological inadequacy continue to this day with hysteria and immaturity being implicated, although an interesting side-line was researched in 1982 on nausea and vomiting in pregnancy in women who already had children with milk allergy. Although they experienced nausea and vomiting at the same rate as mothers with children without milk allergy, they were more likely to have persistent vomiting throughout the day. Twice as many mothers in the allergic group had food aversions.

Jarnfelt-Samisioe and others (1983) did a detailed study of 240 women who had had 948 pregnancies between them and described various details about them. They concluded that the nausea and vomiting was not caused by levels of the human chorionic gonadotrophin. They thought women suffered less with subsequent pregnancies due to maternal adaptation to hormonal changes. They still considered that psychological aspects may play an important role.

Another interesting aspect involving the consequences of diet on nausea and vomiting in pregnancy was done by Minturn and Weiher in 1984. This examined nutritional and cultural variables in a large study across societies listed in Murdock's and White's standard cross-cultural samples and Human Relation Area files. Eighty-three societies had some information on pregnancy sickness, food cravings and taboos. All geographic areas were represented in a final total of thirty-one societies. It transpired that pregnancy sickness is not a universal symptom and that women in those societies who ate green vegetables and fats more regularly were less likely to have it. Those whose staple diet was maize did not appear to suffer from it. Otherwise no correlations were found across societies with geographic variables, food taboos or cravings. The authors suggested that those who attributed nausea and vomiting to psychological causes may have over-emphasised them.

Later studies looked at the people who suffered with nausea and vomiting and tried to discover links between them and consequent causes. Conflicting results ensued. Further theories were advanced regarding slow adaptation to the increased hormonal load on the liver (Jarnfelt-Samsioe, *et al.*, 1986) and differences in adrenal activity and renal excretion of metabolites. Psychic factors were falling from favour. Dilorio (1985) recognised that resting was very helpful and wondered whether there was a link with orthostatic hypertension (blood pressure falling when you stand up).

Further studies analysed increasing numbers of women, including one study with 7767 mothers who had been pregnant during a period of malathion spraying, (Pettitti, 1986). They looked particularly at those who had miscarried, and found that the risk of miscarriage was higher in those who were not nauseated, but there was no association between stillbirth and nausea and vomiting in pregnancy. It was theorised that levels of human chorionic gonadotrophin, progesterone and oestrogen could explain the symptoms. The authors thought that sickness was easier to tolerate if it was regarded as a physical rather than mental symptom, and as a sign of fetal health.

Depue *et al.* (1987) also considered high levels of oestrogen in early pregnancy to be the cause. Women who are pregnant for the first time, and heavy women, have higher circulating levels of oestrogen and are more likely to be sick. Oestriol concentrations were 26% higher in white women diagnosed as having *hyperemesis gravidarum*. Whitehead *et al.* (1992) thought that the sickness might be due to an action of hormones on the area postrema, a circumventricular organ on the floor of the fourth ventricle situated outside the blood-brain barrier.

It is generally known as the chemoreceptor trigger zone, involved not only with emesis (vomiting), but also with taste aversions, the anorexic effect of tumours, energy balance and other functions (Borison, 1989). The taste aversion activity of this area of the brain is not only associated with sickness but with altered taste perceptions (Hook, 1978).

As yet no cause has been conclusively identified, although with increasing amounts of research it may well be. Effective and safe treatment must be dependent on identifying the cause beyond reasonable doubt.

· *Maureen* ·

I only had it with my second son Jonathan [Maureen also has a daughter] *and then I was sick even before it occurred to me that I could be pregnant as I had just had a miscarriage and a D & C.*

I felt sick all day, every day, apart from ten days. I would lie on the sofa watching Postman Pat, Button Moon and Rainbow over and over again because it kept Anthony quiet. I felt I short-changed him because I wasn't able to do anything with him.

I was even lying on the operating table about to have my elective caesarean when I said 'I'm sorry – I need a bowl.' It went instantly though, the moment I had him.

I think it's hormonal. Before I had Anthony I used to have very bad headaches, but while I was pregnant with him I didn't have any. With Jonathan I had to have migraine treatment while I was pregnant because the headaches were so bad.

Chapter Seven

EVERYDAY REMEDIES

To some extent pregnancy sickness can be improved by taking simple everyday measures. It is worth thinking about them, even if they seem difficult or impossible, because you may be able to help yourself. The inertia and lassitude that often accompany early pregnancy can make it hard to find the energy to change things and you may drift on feeling ill unnecessarily, because you haven't the strength to alter your daily pattern.

It might be helpful to look at your lifestyle with your partner or a friend to see where you can improve matters. You may have to abandon some of the things that you normally enjoy, until you feel better. All the suggestions included here have helped someone at some time, and can often be managed even when you don't want to reveal your pregnancy at work or to family and friends yet.

· *Things to Do* ·

More rest

Many women have reported a link between their pregnancy sickness and tiredness. Overwhelming tiredness is a symptom of early pregnancy which often takes people by surprise. Many find it hard to believe that what is still a very tiny fetus can make them feel quite so exhausted.

It can of course be very difficult to get extra rest or sleep, either at work or if you are at home with children. Although it may seem indulgent or unnecessary, resting with your feet up and head slightly elevated is often described as the one thing that made the biggest difference to nausea and vomiting in pregnancy. Women with very severe vomiting problems describe having to keep absolutely still in order to retain food.

You may need to go to bed several hours before your normal bedtime. You may also find it useful to share children's nap times, hard though it is to give up the chance to get on with something. If you can manage this, you will find it easier to sleep if you unplug the phone or put on the answering machine and muffle the doorbell. You may have to think hard about your priorities and appreciate that although pregnancy seems to stretch ahead for a long while, the time that you may need to take these steps for is comparatively short.

Get up slowly

Take time about getting out of bed and get ready for the day gradually. It can be really helpful to have tea and toast brought to you in bed, but if that is not possible, have an air-tight tin of biscuits or crackers by your bedside, with a thermos full of boiled water to make a herbal tea before putting a foot out of bed. Little cartons of fruit juice that can be drunk through a straw are useful to sip during the night or first thing in the morning.

Indulge your cravings

In fact it is hard not to indulge cravings, but you may feel guilty about a passion for food that seems unhealthy. Unless it's obviously toxic, you should find that a little, or even a lot, of what you fancy makes you feel better.

Get plenty of exercise and fresh air

This is easier said than done if you feel you are dragging yourself about, or if your fresh air is traffic-polluted. However, a walk in the park, or a brisk walk to work or to collect children from school, or somewhere for a purpose, can stimulate the endorphins – the body's natural painkillers – and make you feel better. You may find that walking, swimming or cycling a certain distance each day improves the way you feel.

Separate drinks and meals

If you sip drinks between meals, instead of with them, you are less likely to vomit. Some people find that delaying the first drink of the day as long as possible is helpful.

Drinks

Fizzy drinks such as carbonated water, ginger ale, ginger beer or lemonade drunk slowly can all help, particularly if a build-up of gas in your stomach is contributing to the feeling of nausea. Otherwise try weak tea with or without milk, lemon barley water hot or cold, hot water with a slice of lemon in it, Bovril, very cold or hot milk, herb teas (see p. 89) or instant fennel drink. You could also try a cup of hot water with a teaspoon of cider vinegar in it.

Meals

See Chapter Eight for suggestions about what to eat. Try eating little and often: small sandwiches every two hours if larger meals make you sick or you cannot face preparing them. Try having your food either very hot or very cold.

After meals – Sit upright, don't slouch.

Between meals – You may like to suck ice chips, or ice cubes made with water, juice or herb tea (see p. 89). Ice lollies can also be welcome.

Take vitamin supplements or increase your intake of foods rich in vitamin B6, potassium, magnesium, folic acid, etc. (see pp. 68–70).

Sweets

Boiled sweets or mints can be invaluable in preventing sickness. If you suck them slowly they can reduce nausea and disguise the metallic taste in the mouth that often accompanies it. It may be better to avoid those which are highly coloured. You will be able to identify the type that will help you most. Those that have been recommended by other women include lemon, aniseed, liquorice, glucose and ginger. Chewing gum may help too.

Get more help from your partner

It can be very difficult to fully comprehend exactly how ill another person is feeling, so it may be useful for your partner to read this book or talk to other women who have experienced morning sickness. If he sympathises and realises that his help can make it more tolerable for you, you may well feel better.

Other suggested remedies

- Remedies to restore your *electrolyte balance* after vomiting are available from a chemist (e.g. *Dioralyte*) but you can make a drink at home that serves the same purpose. Mix half a teaspoon salt and half a teaspoon honey in a pint of warm water. Take it very slowly: one teaspoon every 15 minutes for the first hour, two teaspoons every 15 minutes for the next hour and three teaspoons every 15 minutes after that. This won't sustain you for long but, according to Lisa Goldstein, it will stay down (Goldstein, 1996).
- Try *lemon* therapy; sniff them, rub them on your hand, suck or bite into them or drink the juice – you might even try just thinking about them.
- Try eating a *grape* or two every hour (Korte, 1995). Chewing dried papaya also helps some people.
- Try one *milk of magnesia* tablet 2–3 times a day between meals (see p. 77).
- *Fructose:* Add fruit sugar (available in health food stores) to drinks

if all you can manage is liquids. It provides a sustained release of energy rather than the peak followed by trough that you get with glucose.

- Try *gripe water* in recommended doses. It no longer contains alcohol in this country although it is available in the original formula in Ireland.
- Take a tiny amount of *gin*. Half a teaspoon can be beneficial in relieving a build-up of gas leading to nausea. It is safe for pregnant women to drink up to 8 units of alcohol per week in divided amounts (1 unit of alcohol being half a pint of ordinary strength beer, a small glass of wine or a single measure of spirits).

There are also a number of steps that you can take to avoid aggravating or stimulating nausea and vomiting. Clearly avoidance can be very difficult to practise, particularly in work situations or when travelling. It may be possible with forethought though to devise new patterns of doing things so that you need not face up to the ones that make you feel worst. Some may be caused by habits that can be broken.

· *Things to Avoid* ·

- Avoid cooking or eating greasy or *fried foods* which are hard to digest and often nauseating to pregnant women.
- Avoid drinks containing *caffeine*, such as coffee, cola, tea, all of which can make you feel sick. Many people go off them anyway.
- Avoid *cooking* if possible, pregnancy is often the cue for a father to improve his cooking skills. Some women cannot bear the smell but are happy to eat cooked food: others can only tolerate uncooked food such as fruit, vegetables, cereals and sandwiches.
- Avoid *brushing your teeth* immediately after meals. Teeth brushing can be very problematic for some people, merely putting the tooth-brush into their mouths causes them to gag. You may have to delay teeth cleaning to your best time of day, perhaps shortly before eating. Dental hygiene can be difficult, particularly if sweets are the only things to quell your nausea. Gums are more inclined to bleed and are more susceptible to infection due to the action of progesterone, even when you can brush them regularly. Try a mouthwash if it is impossible to brush.
- Avoid *sudden movements*, especially just after getting up. Allowing double the time to get ready can help. Vertigo or giddiness is often a sign of early pregnancy so that you may get a feeling of having missed your footing. It doesn't generally last past the first weeks but

can contribute to nausea. Low blood sugar can also give you a weak and giddy feeling – eating or sucking sweets will help if you can manage it. Fructose sweets may work best.

- *Bad smells* such as drains, rubbish and animal excreta are normally nauseating and intended to put us off. In pregnancy they may be doubly repugnant, so too may other smells that are noxious, such as cigarette smoke or exhaust fumes. Less explicably smells like perfume, even your own, or the smell of food can be revolting. If you come across something you will just have to hold your breath and rush past, but if the trouble is caused by your pets, or people around you smoking, you will just have to be blunt about the way it affects you. In any case, pregnant women should avoid emptying cat trays because of the slight risk of contracting toxoplasmosis from their animals. Passive smoking in pregnancy is thought to lead to an increase in the risk of cot death.

- Avoid wearing *tight clothing* or clothes with tight waistbands You may find that clothing becomes tight around the waist very early in pregnancy, long before the pregnancy could be expected to show. This can be caused by hormone changes similar to those which result in the abdominal distension some women experience before a period. Your breasts, too, may not only become tender but larger too, long before the birth, so that you may need to buy bigger sizes fairly early on. It can be quite hard to accept that your clothes are too tight, especially early on when you are only just getting used to being pregnant and don't want to have to buy or wear maternity clothes yet. However, squeezing into your normal clothes can put uncomfortable pressure on your stomach and exacerbate nausea. Loose clothes or elasticated waistbands can help.

- Avoid routine *iron preparations* if blood tests show you do not need them. Some iron tablets, at one time prescribed routinely for pregnant women, can cause nausea and constipation in some people. Evidence suggests that many women do not need them because the body is designed to cope with a degree of anaemia in pregnancy. Blood and iron is not lost through menstruation and your blood volume is greater in pregnancy, so that the need for supplementation is not as great as was formerly thought.

In fact, there is some evidence to suggest that women with adequate haemoglobin levels (11g or above) should not have additional iron as high levels can increase the chance of postpartum haemorrhage and make the red cells bigger so that they cannot cross the placenta.

If, however, you are one of the 7% or so of women who need extra iron and feel better with it, but your iron tablets make you feel sick, ask for a change of preparation. You can get capsules on prescription, with contents that are time-released and so absorbed gradually, either from your doctor or midwife, or over the counter (e.g. *Fefol* spansules available from chemists which provide iron and folic acid). Alternatively you can try *Floradix*, a liquid iron preparation, also available in tablet form, which is made from iron-rich herbs and is available in health food shops and chemists. It is useful for women who have difficulty in tolerating other forms of iron, although more expensive than *Fefol*. (See p. 69 for a list of foods rich in iron.)

- Avoid travelling by car. This can be difficult although there may be ways around it such as walking, cycling or public transport. Many sickness sufferers are often better if they are driving or at least sitting in the front. On the other hand, if you are afraid that you will be sick, you may prefer the comparative privacy of the car to being sick more publicly. It helps to keep airline sick bags (see p. 119), or a bucket lined with a bin liner, in the car.

If car travel is particularly difficult you may need to limit it to the absolute minimum for the time being and avoid any journey that is not strictly necessary.

· *Eirlys Penn* ·

I felt nauseous from week five onwards, but was not actually sick except once at 13 weeks when I had assumed it would be over. However I did spend three months on our chaise longue feeling sorry for myself. I couldn't get into the kitchen so my husband took up cooking with enthusiasm and fortunately still is. I couldn't stand strong smells like dill but did find that I craved salty foods such as crisps, and bland stodgy things like baked potatoes which I liked best.

In the end what seemed to cure it was cycling. I knew Libby Purves recommends getting out and taking your mind off it in one of her books, and it turned out to be true. My cycling husband took me off to Yorkshire and I found I had to really pedal hard to keep up with him because he is a much fitter cyclist than me.

Oddly enough the holiday cured my nausea. I don't know whether it was the clean air, the copious food (big B & B breakfasts) or the exercise. Maybe it was just being distracted that helped. Anyway, my only bad moment was brushing my teeth; poking the toothbrush at my molars would make me gag.

· *Claire* ·

Last time I had dreadful nausea from five weeks right until after the birth, although I was better for a spell at about 20 weeks. However, I was only sick a few times because I was able to control it by eating. I would really have to fancy something though; my husband found it frustrating because it was never the same thing, it changed almost from day to day. However, if I could eat in the first few minutes after waking I would be OK. I used to eat a cooked breakfast – bacon, eggs, fried bread – and then perhaps a cheese sandwich an hour-and-a-half later. Constant nibbling seems to stave it off. Someone suggested not drinking very much and that seemed to help. I only drink fizzy water and lemonade anyway, I've gone off tea and coffee (I am currently 13 weeks pregnant).

I'm lucky in a way, being a GP, because I can organise my own work to a certain extent. I can delay calling my next patient while I eat a couple of crisps or have a sip of lemonade. If I feel really awful I can share out my work load with my partners. I think it would be more difficult if I was working in hospital, working for a boss. I do find it better at work when my mind is taken off it, rather than being at home thinking about it. I'm better off outside walking in the fresh air too.

I do eat constantly. I put on about a stone in the first three months last time although it eased off later. The nausea is possibly marginally better this time, but it is much worse when I am tired. Although I am working part-time this time as I've got an eighteen-month-old to look after, I feel much better with a good rest and if I sleep well. I try to go to bed at the same time as he does.

Smells are bad – we've got a cupboard with onions in that really makes me retch if it is opened. If the burping and belching are bad in the evening, making me feel sick, I sometimes have a sip of sherry which seems to help although I'm not sure why – perhaps it relaxes something. I don't think I could get ginger near my mouth.

Last time it lasted right into labour – I was being dreadfully sick while I was in labour although they tried some medication. Fortunately that worked and so I had some energy left for labour.

The nausea finally wore off about two days after the birth, it was wonderful to actually be hungry again and to look forward to food with pleasure rather than something to be eaten immediately to stop the nausea.

My partner says that if men had babies they would have found a cure a long time ago.

Several weeks later Claire was feeling much better.

Chapter Eight

DIETARY CHANGES

Feeling sick or vomiting are usually linked to eating something that disagrees with you. It seems logical that your diet in pregnancy may affect you in the same way. In fact this is not necessarily the case; you may be sickened by anything, food you normally enjoy and conversely find yourself longing for, while tolerating something that would not appeal to you were you not pregnant. In an ideal world, women would eat well *before* pregnancy, taking a folic acid and perhaps a multivitamin supplement before conceiving, then eating nutritious, well-balanced meals throughout pregnancy, without gaining excessive weight.

In reality, even those who have prepared themselves well may find that they cannot tolerate anything except what they consider junk foods. They consume sweets and little else, vomiting the nutritious foods they do eat and either failing to gain weight, or eating stodgy foods constantly to stave off nausea or ravenous constant hunger, thus gaining weight alarmingly rapidly. It can be hard to credit that what is still a minute fetus can be having such an impact on your body.

Of all these dietary changes, perhaps the one that causes the greatest concern is the fear that the baby will be starved of nutrients and suffer as a consequence. In fact a fetus is well adapted to satisfy all its needs from the mother and only in very extreme cases does vomiting or inability to eat have a deleterious effect on the baby. In fact nausea and vomiting are so common as almost to be normal; if it affected babies adversely it would be a major design fault – you may feel that morning sickness itself falls into that category! Interestingly, recent research does suggest a rationale for the condition (Godfrey *et al.*, 1996). It is apparently usual for sheep farmers to put sheep on to rich grazing land around the time they are mated. They eat a good diet prior to pregnancy and then they are put on poor pasture for the early part of pregnancy as high nutrient levels in early pregnancy can suppress placental, and therefore fetal, growth.

It has been observed that women who eat high carbohydrate meals in early pregnancy give birth to babies of lower birthweight, with smaller placentas, which are generally held to be less favourable indicators of health in newborn babies. It may be that this phenomenon goes some way to explaining the existence of nausea and vomiting in pregnancy, although not perhaps why some women are able to eat high carbohydrate diets without difficulty.

Perhaps the most difficult thing is finding food that is appealing and does not need much preparation. For many women cooking is completely unthinkable. If your partner will prepare food for you, it can make eating much more acceptable. If nothing seems to appeal to you at the moment, try reading the lists of food that some people find palatable while they are feeling sick. There may be something that you have not thought of which sparks your appetite at the moment.

It is thought that morning sickness may be caused by deficiencies of particular vitamins and minerals and that vomiting further depletes reserves causing a vicious circle (Czeizel *et al.*, 1992) (see *Vitamin and Mineral Therapy* p. 73). If this might apply to you it may be worth taking vitamin and mineral supplements initially to restore the balance, and then, if your condition improves and you are able to keep food down, eat foods that are rich in such vitamins and minerals, particularly vitamin B, magnesium and zinc (see pp. 68–70).

Some substances, particularly ginger or lemons, can be considered either part of your diet or a herbal remedy. Ginger's particular efficacy earns it a special mention (see p.71). It is also worth trying eating *umeboshie* or *ume plums* from a health food shop.

Although it may feel self-indulgent or childish, it may be useful to consider eating baby food. Most baby foods available commercially are fortified with vitamins and are designed to be easily digested. You might like to consider rusks, dehydrated meals in packets, purées or jars, or the instant fennel drink. If it seems extravagant, think of it going direct to the baby. Alternatively, invalid or convalescent foods contain essential vitamins and minerals too and can be useful if you can keep them down. Gruel, an invalid food with a long tradition, can be made by adding 2 tablespoons medium oatmeal to a pint of water and leaving it to stand overnight. Next day, strain off the oatmeal and boil the remaining liquid until it is reduced by half. Add sugar, salt, milk or lemon juice to taste.

Obviously you will have to be guided by how you feel and what help is available to you. Something that helps one woman may seem revolting to another: something that helps now, may repel you in a couple of days. However, there is some evidence that it can help to eat small carbohydrate-rich meals frequently, at least every two hours. Sandwiches which can be prepared in advance by someone else may be useful, especially if they are filled with whatever appeals to you, even if it is a bit unusual.

Bland Foods High in Carbohydrate

Rice

Baked potato

Pasta

Crackers

Biscuits

Baby rusks

Baby cereals

Hot cereals – porridge

Gruel

Breakfast cereals

Dry toast

Toast (no butter) and jam

Baked beans on toast

Soup and toast

Scones

Oat cakes

Rice cakes

Bananas

Milk – hot or cold

Yoghurt

Fromage frais

Sandwiches – vary the type of bread and try the following fillings

Marmite

Cheese

Pickle

Egg

Ham

Chicken

Turkey

Cottage Cheese

Peanut Butter

Prawns

Tuna

Sardine

Smoked Mackerel

Tomato

Banana

Beetroot

Cucumber

Grated carrot

Grated apple

Foods Rich in Magnesium

Spinach

Swiss Chard

Kale

Nuts

Pumpkin seeds

Sunflower seeds

Avocado

Beans – kidney, navy, pinto, lima, soya

Broccoli

Tofu

Cereals

Wheat germ

Peanuts and peanut butter

Shrimps

Foods Rich in Potassium

Dried apricots

Bananas

Melon

Dates

Dried figs

Prunes

Raisins

Water melon

Fruit juices – apricot, grapefruit,
   orange, pineapple, prune, tomato

Broccoli

Cooked dried beans

Peanuts

Potatoes

Spinach

Squash (yellow and orange)

Yams

Foods Rich in Iron

Red meat (liver not
  recommended)
Lean meat – especially kidney
Wheatgerm
Watercress
Dried fruit – prunes, apricots,
  raisins
Celeriac
Butter beans
Kidney beans

Dark green vegetables
Cream
Cottage cheese
Cocoa
Molasses
Nettles
Parsley
Dandelion
Alfalfa
Shellfish

Foods Rich in Zinc

Ginger
Lamb chops
Seafood – prawns, oysters
Wholewheat
Bran
Leafy vegetables
Brazil nuts
Non-fat dried milk

Egg yolk
Rye
Oats
Peanuts
Watercress
Corn
Rice bran

Foods Rich in Vitamin B6

Sesame seeds
Chick peas
Wheat bran
Baked potato with skin
Bananas
Rye flour (dark)
Mackerel
Molasses
Brewer's yeast (see p. 70).
Plantain
Salmon
Coconut
Sweet corn

Dried sunflower seeds
All-Bran cereal
Wheat germ
Hazelnuts
Chicken liver
Beef steaks
Prune juice
Chicken
Corn flour
Turkey (dark meat)
Raisins
Spinach

If you take a vitamin B6 supplement it is better taken as part of a
B-complex rather than alone: you should not take a high dosage tablet.
If you do take vitamin B taper off gradually after your baby is born: if
you stop it suddenly you may get rebound deficiency symptoms.

Food Rich in Folic Acid

Green leafy vegetables
Brussels sprouts
Broccoli
Spinach
Fortified bread

Breakfast cereals
Oranges
Bananas
Avocado
Marmite

Drinks

Milk – hot or very cold
Fizzy drinks – lemonade,
    ginger beer or ale,
    soda or tonic water
Still or fizzy water
Fruit juices – apple, mango,
    orange, grape, pineapple.
    For a drink rich in iron and
    vitamin B6 try 1 tsp each
    of Brewer's yeast and
    wheatgerm mixed with
    fruit juice.

Weak tea
Squashes and cordials
Herb teas

Fruit and Nuts

Apples – raw or stewed
Bananas
Oranges
Grapefruit
Tangerines
Satsumas
Plums

Peaches
Pears
Blackcurrants
Melons
Strawberries
Nuts

Vegetables

Raw carrots
Celery
Peas
Mashed potato
Soups
Cabbage

Lettuce
Radishes
Brussels sprouts
Watercress
Broccoli

· *Ginger* ·

Ginger crosses the boundary between being an everyday remedy and a herbal treatment because it is a culinary herb, used both fresh and in its dried powdered form. It has a particular place in treating nausea and vomiting, not only in pregnancy but with travel and other kinds of sickness too. Several of the women who tell their story in this book have found it helpful and it is certainly worth a try.

Of 30 women suffering from *hyperemesis gravidarum* who took part in a double blind trial (Fischer-Rasmussen *et al.*, 1990) with randomised cross-over, taking either 250mg of ginger or 250mg of lactose (milk sugar) contained in a capsule four times a day, were asked which seemed to relieve their symptoms most, nineteen preferred ginger, 4 preferred the placebo and 4 could not state a preference. Objective scores of relief of symptoms showed significantly greater relief with the ginger and no side-effects were observed. The amount they consumed was no more than would be found in ginger cakes or tarts and was thought to have no ill effect on the babies.

A much higher dose recommended to Kathryn Butler of 940mg worked temporarily but left her with a spicy burning indigestion that lasted for hours and meant she was unwilling to try it again. However, she states that mothers writing in to *Womenwise* (an American publication) found doses as high as 10–12 capsules an hour more effective than *Dramamine* (an over-the-counter travel sickness remedy) in preventing nausea and sickness.

Ginger is thought to work in several ways. It improves motility in the gastrointestinal tract itself, so that food passes more rapidly through the digestive system and is less likely to cause nausea and vomiting. It is also considered to have absorbent properties which may reduce the stimuli to the chemoreceptor area of the brain which sends messages to the emetic centre, prompting nausea and vomiting. The messages can be initiated by toxic substances and also by raised blood levels of urea and ketones (Fischer-Rasmussen *et al.* 1990). Ginger may also block the gastrointestinal reactions and subsequent nausea feedback. It is thought to work on the level of the central nervous system (Mowrey & Clayson, 1982). Most interestingly, it is one of the richest food sources of zinc.

Ways to take Ginger

Drinks

Ginger beer or ale

Infusion of ginger-like tea. Pour boiling water on to dried ginger root or fresh grated root. Pieces of lemongrass added to the infusion can help. Allow to stand for 15 minutes. Sweeten with honey if wanted. The tea can be mixed with chamomile and frozen into cubes.

Instant ginger drink available from oriental food shops.

Fresh ginger root

This is used in cooking in savoury dishes.

Dried ginger

This can be used in cakes, biscuits or taken as capsules (250mg four times a day), available from chemists, health food shops or Baldwin's (see p. 119).

Crystallised ginger

This is available in pieces at grocers or health food shops.

Ginger marmalade

This can be spread on toast, or stirred into porridge.

Biscuits

A further way of incorporating ginger into your diet is described in Catherine Lewis's *Good Food Before Birth* (Unwin, 1984) now unfortunately out of print. If you can face cooking or can get someone to do it for you, try her recipe for Ginger Root Snaps.

Ginger Root Snaps

340g/12oz wholewheat flour
1 tablespoon ginger powder
1 tablespoon grated root ginger
2 tablespoons chopped preserved ginger or candied peel.
50g/2oz muscovado or demerara sugar
225g/8oz black treacle or molasses
80g/3oz butter or whey-free margarine
A little milk or soya milk to mix.

1. Preheat oven to 325°F/150°C/Gas mark 3.
2. Mix the dry ingredients in a bowl.
3. Heat the butter and when just melted stir in the treacle or molasses and mix well.
4. Add to the dry ingredients and knead to a paste, adding a little milk. The more milk you add the softer the biscuits will be.

Without milk they will be very hard, 1–2 tablespoons should be enough.

5. Shape into walnut-sized pieces.
6. Place on a greased baking sheet and flatten.
7. Bake for 30 minutes.

· *Vitamin and Mineral Therapy* ·

The best way of ensuring that your baby will receive all the vitamins and minerals it needs for healthy growth is to eat well. In this way you will start your pregnancy with good reserves of all the essential nutrients including folic acid and all should continue to go well throughout the pregnancy. However, although this should be your aim, and it is certainly a better idea than eating any old thing and hoping to redress the balance with a multivitamin, there can be reasons why you may not achieve it, pregnancy sickness being just one of them.

Folic acid

If you are planning pregnancy you are recommended by the Department of Health (1994) to consume 400mcg of folic acid each day to reduce the risk of having a baby with neural tube defects such as spina bifida and anencephaly. It is not easy to obtain this amount from food sources, which include green leafy vegetables such as Brussels sprouts, broccoli, spinach, fortified breads and breakfast cereals, oranges, bananas, avocados, and Marmite. Taking folic acid prior to pregnancy has been shown to reduce the chance of a baby being born with neural tube defects by as much as 72%. A 400mcg tablet is available on prescription or over the counter and should be taken every day for at least a month prior to conception and until you are 14 weeks pregnant.

Vitamins

Folic acid supplementation is recommended, but should you also take a multivitamin? Experts disagree on this: some feel that most women eat more than enough to prevent any nutritional deficiency and that not everything is known about the need for vitamins, or whether taking extra could cause long-term problems in babies. There may be as yet undiscovered value in eating well rather than taking supplements, and that vitamins and minerals from food sources are better absorbed by the body.

Other experts have produced evidence to show that taking vitamins around the time of conception not only reduces the likelihood of having a damaged baby but also reduces the chances of your having nausea, vomiting and vertigo in pregnancy. Moreover, some contend that vomiting, not surprisingly, can lead to vitamin and mineral deficiencies. If these are treated by giving supplements then the cycle of vomiting – deficiency – feeling worse – vomiting can be broken.

Vitamin B6

Vitamin B6 (pyridoxine) in a dosage of 25mg orally every 8 hours for 72 hours has been shown to have a significant effect in reducing nausea and vomiting in women with severe pregnancy sickness symptoms. A double blind randomised control trial of 59 women showed that it helped to stop those whose nausea and vomiting symptoms rated more that seven on a scale of 0–10, but that it was no more effective than the placebo for those who were not so badly affected. (Sahakian *et al.*, 1991).

The maximum recommended dosage in pregnancy is 100mg daily (National Academy of Science, 1989) and is best taken as a B-complex tablet. (See p. 69 for dietary ways of increasing your vitamin B6 intake.)

Vitamin B deficiency is known to be a cause of anxiety and depression and general malaise as well as nausea and loss of appetite, so correcting a deficiency might make you feel better as well as improving your other symptoms.

Czeizel *et al.* (1992), who have done a lot of work relating to vitamin supplementation and reproduction, did a trial with 1000 Hungarian women who were planning pregnancy. A group of 500 were given a vitamin supplement containing:

Vitamin A	6000IU	Ca-Pantothenate	10mg
Vitamin B1	1.6mg	Biotin	0.2mg
Vitamin B2	1.8mg	Calcium	125mg
Vitamin B6	2.6mg	Phosphorus	125mg
Vitamin B12	4.0mcg	Magnesium	100mg
Vitamin C	100mg	Iron	60mg
Vitamin D	500IU	Copper	1mg
Vitamin E	15mg	Manganese	1mg
Nicotinamide	19mg	Zinc	7.5mg

The other 500 were given a placebo containing:

Vitamin C	7.5mg	Manganese	1mg
Copper	1mg	Zinc	7.5mg

Both groups took the tablets for a minimum of a month before conception. Both groups reported nausea and vomiting in early pregnancy. Significantly fewer women in the multi-vitamin group suffered from nausea and vomiting (3.4% as opposed to 7.4%) and the researchers speculated that, as the vitamin B-complex dose was low, this was due to generally improved nutritional status and metabolism. The percentage of sufferers was very low in both groups, which raises the question of whether the zinc that they *all* took had a beneficial effect.

Zinc

Zinc requirements increase during pregnancy and adequate dietary zinc is thought to be essential during pregnancy and lactation for the development of an intact immune system. One study found that pregnant and breast-feeding mothers were consuming only 42% of the Recommended Daily Allowance (15–19 mg per day). Those on calorie-restricted diets and with anorexia take in even less. One study of pregnant women described as lean (of a Body Mass Index of less than 19.8 kg/m – for example, someone of 5ft 5ins who weighed under eight and a half stone), who were given zinc supplements in pregnancy, had babies nearly half a kilogram heavier than was expected. Also, there was a 50 per cent reduction in premature births (Goldenberg, 1996). The authors of this study recommend that women intending to become pregnant, or already pregnant, should take a zinc supplement as routinely as folic acid.

Vegetarians are particularly likely to be zinc-deficient for two reasons. One is that they do not eat meat, poultry and seafood which are the best sources of dietary zinc, but also because plant foods contain phytic acid. This binds with zinc and other minerals to form phytates – insoluble compounds which cannot be absorbed by the body and so are excreted, reducing the availability of the zinc consumed. Vegans and lacto-vegetarians are more at risk than those who eat eggs, vegans being particularly at risk (Freeland-Graves *et al.*, 1980). Vegetarian foods that are richest in zinc include cheese, wholegrains and legumes.

If you do take a zinc supplement, it is important to avoid taking it at the same time as any of the following food or drink, as they may prevent the zinc being absorbed: soya protein isolates, soya base milk foods, coffee, cow's milk, cheese, hamburgers, celery, lemon, brown bread, iron supplements, wholewheat bread, high-fibre foods and bran. (Stewart & Davies, 1987). Blackmore's *Bio-Zinc* is easy on the stomach and contains vitamins A and B6 as well.

It is interesting to note that ginger, which so many women find useful in treating pregnancy sickness, is very rich in zinc, and that societies whose staple diet is maize, which is also a good source of dietary zinc, do not experience pregnancy sickness. Zinc deficiency can result in impairment of the senses of taste and smell, which as the stories show are common in women with pregnancy sickness. White flecks on the finger nails, commonly attributed to calcium deficiency, are in fact due to a lack of zinc (Stewart & Davies, 1987).

· *Jackie Cowhig* ·

By the time I was five months pregnant with my third child I was still feeling absolutely dreadful – sea-sick all the time. I could barely eat and felt really unbalanced all day. The nausea came in waves and nothing seemed to help – neither eating or not eating. It was very unpredictable; sometimes it was worse than at other times and it made it very difficult to cope with my two small children. I was also anaemic which didn't help.

I tried Sea-Bands but they only helped very slightly. Zinc was suggested and I tried it. By the end of the first week of taking it there was some improvement and after two weeks I felt much better. Provided I take it at opposite ends of the day from the iron, it seems to have helped where nothing else has. I'm sure it's not coincidence.

· *Suzanna Miller* ·
(currently 36 weeks pregnant)

My worst symptom has been excessive salivation – ptyalism. It is so bad that I have to keep a cup with me all the time. I was also getting awful heartburn which would make me retch. Zinc was suggested as a long shot seven weeks ago and although my symptoms have not gone, they are greatly improved. My appetite has increased and I'm now eating quite a lot. The food is going down and not just sitting there. I mainly drink water; anything else like tea or Coca Cola is not a good idea as it irritates the system but now I can manage some milk towards the end of the day.

Although I still have to sleep propped up on pillows, I don't wake up with acid heartburn any longer and I am much less likely to retch. It has definitely made a difference – it was the best bit of advice so far.

Caroline Wilson (see p. 77) is currently expecting her fourth child and has been taking zinc since the start of pregnancy. At the time of writing she has not been sick and she is now past the six-weeks-two-days stage when she started vomiting in all her previous pregnancies.

Chloride

Salting food to taste can replace lost chloride and in fact salty food often seems desirable when you've been sick, but excessive salt is best avoided.

Magnesium

Magnesium stores are diminished by vomiting and magnesium deficiency can exacerbate nausea. Moreover, uncorrected magnesium deficiency may impair repletion of cellular potassium (Whang *et al.*, 1992). You can help to replace it by chewing or sucking one *milk of magnesia* tablet 2–3 times a day (Newman *et al.*, 1993). It both soothes the stomach and increases the magnesium levels. Each tablet provides 131mg of elemental magnesium. The recommended dose in pregnancy is 320mg (National Academy of Sciences, 1989).

If you wish to take supplements before or during pregnancy, a recommended regime would be:

1 multi-vitamin
1 vitamin B-complex (not a high or mega dose)
1 g vitamin C
3 dolomite tablets (calcium and magnesium)
15mg zinc

Vegans and vegetarians should be taking 3–4 mcgs of vitamin B12 daily, even if they take no other supplement.

It is important not to take more than 7,500–10,000ius of vitamin A daily as higher levels have been associated with malformations in babies. If you take supplements add the vitamin A levels together to make sure they do not exceed this limit.

· Caroline Wilson ·

With Bethany, my first child, I was actually sick first when I was six weeks pregnant, although I felt sick before then. From then on it built up and got gradually worse from being sick three times a day until I was sick as much as 10 or 12 times every single day. It wasn't even a relief, I just felt sick all day. By the time I was 16 weeks pregnant I had to leave work because I was so weak I could hardly stand up. My job was the worst possible, teaching PE and home economics. I had to set them some work and then nip round the corner to the toilets.

Nobody seemed to think it was particularly unusual: the doctor seemed to think it was a typical first pregnancy and that I was being completely dramatic. Eventually he gave me some Avomine *at about 18 weeks, although I was reluctant to take it until I considered the baby had finished developing at about 20 weeks. I took it for a few weeks but it didn't really seem to help.*

The worst thing was the searing headaches that I got and the awful feeling in my throat as if I'd swallowed a tennis ball. I had a terrible burning feeling in my oesophagus and couldn't taste anything. I remember sitting on my bed and sobbing.

For two months I could only eat mashed potato. I was so weak, and couldn't face food so that often all I could do was boil a kettle and mix up instant mashed potato. It stopped about 26 weeks: I think it gradually tailed off so that I was only being sick three times a day again. But then I went straight into indigestion.

With my two boys it wasn't quite so bad. It started earlier (two weeks with Luke) and stopped earlier. With Jesse it started at 4–5 weeks and I was sick 4–5 times a day. I was still being very sick at 17–18 weeks but by the end of the nineteenth week, I was much better, although I don't know why. When I was pregnant with the boys I didn't have any dairy products although I took calcium supplements. This was because Bethany had been sick every day for the first 14 months of her life. She would be sick every night, all over her cot. I used to think she had screamed herself sick for attention but it turned out the poor thing was lactose intolerant. I had had her checked out at six months but the doctor pooh-poohed the idea, although she was sick after every bottle, because she didn't have a rash. Then we got a second opinion and it turned out that she had been screaming with stomach ache.

I'm glad to be remembering this because I'd like another one, and it's good for me to recall how awful it was. My husband can't bear the thought of me being so ill and very tired and irritable. He is reluctant to start again.

Chapter Nine

MEDICAL TREATMENT

Since the *Thalidomide* tragedy, women have been reluctant to take drugs in pregnancy, especially early pregnancy, and doctors are reluctant to prescribe them. This is one reason for writing this book – to provide suggestions of safe, drug-free alternatives to help with the problems of sickness in pregnancy. Not only are women wary of drugs but they may also not be particularly effective. If you are taking tablets to relieve vomiting you may have difficulty in keeping them down long enough to work, and many women who have been ill enough to require them say that they either did not seem to work at all or that they just took the edge off it.

However, if your sickness is so severe that you are considering asking for anti-emetic drugs, you may want to know more about what is on offer and whether taking them will put your baby at risk. There is very little evidence that drugs given to stop pregnancy sickness cause harm, which does not necessarily mean that they do not, just that it seems unlikely that it causes any obvious damage. Moreover, any drawbacks to taking the drugs have to be weighed against the risks involved to the mother and baby if severe sickness continues.

The *British National Formulary* (BNF), a 643-page book written for hospital doctors and pharmacists listing all the available drugs, together with an independent assessment of their value, side-effects and product details states:

> Drugs should be prescribed to the mother only if the expected benefit to the mother is thought to be greater than the risk to the fetus, and all drugs should be avoided if possible in the first trimester. Drugs which have been extensively used in pregnancy and appear to be usually safe should be prescribed in preference to new or untried drugs; and the smallest effective dose should be used. Few drugs have been shown to be teratogenic in man but no drug is safe beyond all doubt in pregnancy.

That statement refers to all drugs, the BNF's guidelines on anti-emetics (drugs to stop vomiting) are as follows: 'Nausea in the first trimester of pregnancy does not require drug therapy. On rare occasions, if vomiting is severe an antihistamine or a phenothiazine (e.g. promethazine) may be required. If symptoms have not settled in 24–48 hours then a specialist opinion should be sought.'

The following includes a list of the drugs and dosages recommended for treating nausea and vomiting in pregnancy when necessary (Lim & Hawkins, 1989):

- *Antihistamines*, such as promethazine hydrochloride (*Phenergan*) and promethazine theoclate (*Avomine*) are recommended in doses of 20–50mg by mouth, with or without 10–20mg pyridoxine hydrochloride (vitamin B6) taken at bedtime.
- *Oral metochlopromide* – (*Maxolon, Metox, Primperan*) at a dose of 10mg three times a day.

Hyperemesis gravidarum, diagnosed by the presence of ketosis, acetonuria and weight loss of at least 5%, and eventual electrolyte imbalance, may be treated by admission to hospital, correction of fluid and electrolyte imbalance, administration of vitamins via a drip, bed rest and sometimes sedation. These sedatives (phenothiazines) might include promethazine (*Phenergan*) 25mg, promazine (*Sparine*) 50 mg, chlorpromazine (*Largactil*) 25–50mg, all of which may be administered via a drip, or prochlorperazine (*Stemetil*) 12.5mg which can be given as an injection three times a day, or given as a suppository.

Antihistamines

The British Medical Journal (see Howden, 1986) says antihistamines are generally recommended for treating nausea and vomiting in pregnancy. Meclozine and cyclizine (*Valloid*) are widely used and appear to be safe. Concern about an association between the use of these drugs and congenital malformations, particularly cleft palate, has not been substantiated in prospective controlled studies (Lewis & Chamberlain, 1982; Fagan & Chadwick, 1983; Nelson & Forfar, 1971). There may however be a weak association between meclozine (*Ancolixin*) and congenital eye defects (Shapiro, Kauffman, Rosenberg *et al.*, 1978). Promethazine may be associated with an increased incidence of congenital hip dislocation (Kullender & Kallen, 1976). Tyack (1991), in a later assessment of vomiting and pregnancy and its treatment, discovered that one study found a lower incidence of birth defects in those mothers who took anti-emetic drugs than those who did not (Kullander & Kallen, 1976), with the exception of the arguable link between promethazine and hip dislocation. He says 'although the safety of antihistamines has not been extensively investigated they are generally regarded as being safe'.

Side-effects on mother – You might experience a dry mouth, blurred vision and drowsiness.

Metochlopromide

Kousen (1993), writing in the *American Family Physician*, suggests that caution is taken with metochlopromide, which although it has been found to be more effective than prochlorperazine or placebo in treating *hyperemisis gravidarum*, has not been used much in pregnancy and has caused problems (acute porphyria – a very rare metabolic disorder) in a mother who took it for several weeks. No associations with congenital malformations have been discovered to date. But Howden (1986) states that it cannot be recommended because of the lack of controlled data.

Side-effects on mother – Side-effects from the low dosages described are very unusual but might include drowsiness, restlessness, diarrhoea, depression, twitching of facial muscles and breast-milk production.

Phenothiazines

Studies have shown both that taking these drugs in early pregnancy cause no congenital malformations and that their incidence may be slightly raised.

Side-effects on mother – Side-effects are similar to those for metochlopromide (Miklovich & Van den Berg, 1976; Slone *et al.*, 1977; Rumeau-Roquette *et al.*, 1977).

This is the evidence as it stands, presented so that you may make up your own mind about the advisability or necessity of taking these particular drugs in early pregnancy. Clearly it would be better to be able to avoid them, but you have to decide for yourself the point at which benefits outweigh the possible risks.

Chapter Ten

ALTERNATIVE THERAPIES

If you have doubts about treating morning sickness with drugs but still want to try and prevent it, you may consider one or more of the alternative medicines.

Not all are thought to be suitable for women in the early weeks of pregnancy; it is unlikely that a reflexologist will treat you then, although it can be a very good method of improving symptoms later in pregnancy. Some homeopaths, too, will not treat women in early pregnancy, although most do, and it is said to be entirely safe (Ford, 1986). Osteopathy may not be useful for treating the symptoms but could be invaluable in repairing the damage to shoulders and spine created by perpetually bending over a lavatory or basin. You may like to start by using some of the suggestions for treating yourself. If they help, but are not the whole answer, or if you feel you need something more powerful, consult a practitioner of whichever therapy appeals to you most. The best way to find one is by word of mouth, but failing that, contact the registers listed at the back of the book. Phone the therapist and find out about whether he or she has experience of treating your problem, how many visits you might need to make and how much it will cost. If you don't feel confident about that person, try someone else.

· *Acupuncture and acupressure* ·

There has been a great deal of interest in the treatment of pregnancy sickness (and other sickness such as that caused by cancer treatments) and the conclusions of at least seven randomised controlled trials of acupressure or acupuncture for pregnancy sickness, is that it works (Vickers, 1996). It may not be effective for everyone (see Sue Parfitt's story p. 111) but it is well worth trying, particularly as you can apply acupressure yourself so it is always readily available. If you find it useful it is possible to buy Sea-Bands or wristlets to apply constant pressure, or hire a TENS machine to stimulate the relevant point (p. 84). Treatment from an acupuncturist is valuable in severe sickness as well as for other pregnancy symptoms.

Acupuncture is a complete system of medicine which was developed in China over 5000 years ago. It is based on the theory that the body consists of two opposing parts – *Yin* and *Yang*. *Yin* is deep, cold and female, *Yang* is hot, stimulating and male. In good health the Yin and Yang are perfectly balanced but in illness the balance is disturbed: the equilibrium can be restored by acupuncture. It is thought that the organs of the body are connected by invisible pathways or meridians. Illness occurs when a meridian or energy pathway becomes obstructed and pain or symptoms may then be felt at any point along the meridian. An acupuncturist will insert very fine needles where the meridian is obstructed and so remove the blockage and allow the vital energy known as *Qi* (pronounced 'chee') to flow freely along the meridians. Free-flowing *Qi* will keep blood circulating, warm the body and fight disease. There are 12 main meridians and more than 365 acupuncture points – the recognised spots where needles may be placed.

The philosophy evolved purely from observing people in ill-health, at a time when doctors were not allowed to do post-mortem examinations on bodies. Everything doctors knew about illness came from observing, questioning and touching their patients. An acupuncturist will pay considerable attention to your appearance, colour and smell as well as what you tell him or her about the way you feel. Your pulse will be particularly informative; a trained acupuncturist can detect 14 different pulses in your wrist, each one providing information about the imbalances within your body. A skilled acupuncturist can even tell the sex of your baby through your pulse.

Traditional Chinese medical diagnoses and descriptions of illness are completely different from Western ones. For example, nausea is attributed to stomach deficiency and three different and distinct pictures of nausea and vomiting in pregnancy are recognised. However, acupuncture is particularly suited to treatment during pregnancy because it is drug free, and quite safe when administered by an experienced, qualified practitioner. Moreover, its scope is far broader than than of Western medicine: it can offer an 80% success rate in turning breech babies, as well as being able to treat such things as varicose veins, sciatica, heartburn, anxiety, haemorrhoids, constipation, migraine, skin rashes, vulval varicosities, sore breasts and abdominal pain (Tiran & Mack, 1995).

Acupressure is the application of deep pressure over acupuncture points. It should work in the same way to relieve obstruction but has the advantage that it can be done at any time, is free, and can be practised whenever symptoms are troublesome. If you are performing it on yourself, you will know when you have found the acupressure point because it will feel tender, more so than the surrounding area. In some cases there may be slight indentations under the skin. Interestingly, Julian Kenyon describes a photographic technique which shows acupuncture points as appearing as electrical pores at the precise spots where the points exist: photographs taken side on to the skin show halos of energy above them (Kenyon, 1987).

The main acupressure point of interest to women suffering from pregnancy sickness is called the Neiquan point, also known as Pericardium 6 or P6. Merely pressing this point, applying pressure to it for ten or more minutes several times a day, has been shown to be effective in reducing nausea, if not vomiting, in 60 pregnant women (Belluomini *et al.*, 1992). Groups were shown how to use acupressure on P6 and on a sham point – the placebo. They applied pressure on the points for 10 minutes each time, four times daily. The researchers, who found, in contrast to others, that nausea got worse with maternal age, also found significant reduction in nausea in the mothers using P6, although it did not affect the number of times they were sick. Other researchers discovered a 60% positive benefit trying continuous acupressure on P6 by means of Sea-Bands which are commercially available wrist bands with a pointed button that is placed over P6, but decided that no particular advantage was to be gained by applying it to both wrists rather than just one. (In this trial Sea-Bands with blunted buttons were used as the placebo.) (De Aloysio & Penacchioni, 1992.)

To apply acupressure to P6 see the diagram on p. 85. P6 is situated three fingers' width down from your first wrist crease and in between your two tendons (measure it with your own fingers). This is two Chinese inches (*cuns*) or thumb-widths up. Push the ball of your thumb lcm deep into the point with pressure in the direction of your hand. There should be some initial discomfort, which will wear off after a while if you maintain pressure at the same intensity. Try this four times a day for at least ten minutes each time. If it seems effective you may want to do it more often; or you could buy some Sea-Bands. These apply constant pressure and were initially designed to prevent seasickness. Another trial found that 75% of women using Sea-Bands improved and 30% seemed to be cured (Hyde, 1989). They do have drawbacks in that they are visible, so may give a clue about your pregnancy if you don't want to admit to it. They can also slip out of place and some people find them uncomfortable. (For details of their availability, see p. 119.)

An alternative way of stimulating P6 is by means of TENS machines, now popular as a means of providing safe, effective and drug-free pain relief in labour. Trials show that a small self-adhesive electrode placed over P6 and attached to a TENS machine is very effective in relieving pregnancy sickness (Evans *et al.*, 1993). It is a bit like having a portable acupuncturist. You may not wish to try it unless your symptoms are severe, but it is possible to hire a small and very discreet TENS unit which can be concealed under your clothes (see p. 118 for details).

If you prefer to have acupuncture for your pregnancy sickness, you will get individual treatment which will help to correct any other underlying imbalance as well. The needles are very fine, about as thick as a hair, and insertion is not usually painful. You may find that you feel slightly light-headed after treatment as your endorphins, your body's natural painkillers, will have been stimulated. Most acupuncturists are happy to treat people in pregnancy but a minority do not. It might be wise to check how long they have been practising and what experience they have of treating your particular symptoms.

In traditional Chinese medical terms there are three categories of pregnancy sickness (Zhao, 1987). The first is 'Rotten and Muddy *Qi* Rebelling Upward due to Pregnancy' in which the treatment lowers the *Qi*, regulates the *Qi* and clears the stomach.

Position of P6

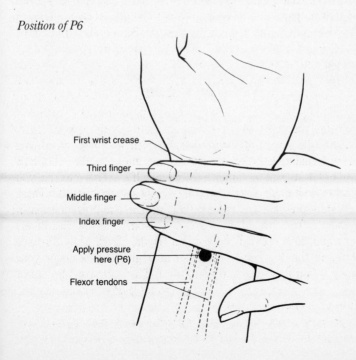

First wrist crease

Third finger

Middle finger

Index finger

Apply pressure
here (P6)

Flexor tendons

The second type is classified as 'Glairy mucus and fluid toxin' which is due to a disturbance of the *Chen Qi* of the *Zang* or solid organs. With this type you would be feeling dizzy, have chest congestion, will vomit a watery substance, have white fur on your tongue and a wiry and sliding pulse (which you will probably not be able to detect).

The third type of morning sickness includes symptoms such as a bitter taste in the mouth, pain in the ribs or hypochondriac region (right side of the ribs underneath the diaphragm) and belching and regurgitation, and a wiry and fast pulse. This is described as 'Rising Fire of the Liver and Gall bladder' and is caused by the *Yin* energy of the kidneys going to the uterus. The liver lacks *Yin*, becomes dried out and the Fire of the Liver burns up and destroys the stomach *Qi*.

Details of acupuncture treatment given to 39 women by Zhao (1987) (described in a comprehensive overview by Beal, 1992) suggest that this treatment will actually stop symptoms. His clients who were described as having, and being treated for, the types of sickness described above, improved within two days of treatment in six cases, within three to five days of treatment in 31 cases, and more than five days in the last case. Clearly it may be inconvenient or costly to go for treatment every day, but it may be worthwhile. A receptionist for two acupuncturists, herself a former sufferer, described seeing women attending with pregnancy sickness and improving with treatment over several days, or a week depending on the severity of the sickness.

· *Natalie Vienes* ·

I have had really bad pregnancy sickness with both my children but it was worse with the second, my daughter. It was so bad that I couldn't get my head off the pillow and had to stay in bed all day, longing to sleep so that I wouldn't be able to feel anything. The only way I can describe it is like someone having a hangover after a really good night out when you have eaten something dodgy as well. I couldn't even keep a sip of water down and had to keep on being admitted to hospital for a week at a time to be rehydrated.

The second time it was even more difficult as it put such a strain on my family who had to look after me. Even my son used to offer me the bucket. Eventually my mother suggested that I went to see an acupuncturist. I had to be taken there and back with a bucket with me in the car. Christine, the acupuncturist, hadn't seen anything like it – I was even being sick as she put the needles in. However, the next two or three hours when I wasn't sick and my bad headache lifted, was heaven. It wasn't a permanent cure though. I would be alright that day and for part of the next, but by the following afternoon I would be back to being sick again. At one time I was having treatment every day.

It cleared up at between seven and eight months and then I started to regain the weight that I had lost rapidly. With my son I went from eight stone to between thirteen and fourteen stone, although it was mostly fluid. I weighed nine stone the day after he was born, and I am normally eight and a half stone. I was sick in labour but recovered quickly after the birth and was able to cope well after a bit more acupuncture.

· *Medical herbalism* ·

Herbs have been used for thousands of years, they are the oldest known form of medicine and they are still used to treat illness by three-quarters of the world's population. The World Health Organisation (WHO) recognises that for many people herbs provide a safe and accessible alternative to imported Western drugs. They are still used alongside mainstream drug treatment in Russia and Germany and in China, where herbs were used as long ago as 2800 BC and where they are still the first line of defence. Herbal medicine is beginning to be appreciated more in the West and is starting to regain popularity.

Specific use of herbs can be particularly useful in early pregnancy when doctors are understandably reluctant to prescribe anti-emetic drugs. They work in several ways to improve nausea and vomiting: they have a beneficial effect on the digestion because they stimulate liver function and improve the tone of the intestinal tract (sluggish progress of food through the digestive system due to the relaxing effect of progesterone on smooth muscle and consequent lowered gastric motility is often considered to be a cause of pregnancy sickness). They also calm and soothe the spasms of an irritable system.

Because herbs are used whole instead of having their active constituents extracted, they are thought to be far safer than drugs made from plant material. Each herb contains within it elements which will counteract the potentially harmful effect of the active part of the plant. For example, dandelion, which acts as a diuretic, also contains within it potassium. Diuretic drugs have to have potassium added to them to replace that lost as a result of the action of the drug on the body.

If your nausea and vomiting is acute it would be wise to consult a qualified medical herbalist (see p. 117 for details) who will be able to tailor a remedy specifically for you, probably incorporating several herbs in a tincture.

If, however, you would like to try some of the gentle herbs which have helped thousands of pregnant women before you, consider some of the following which have been recommended by herbalists with experience of treating morning sickness successfully.

The boundary between herbs used everyday in cooking and ones used as medicines is artificial, as some, such as ginger or coriander, may fall into both categories. It is unlikely that you would use any culinary herb in such quantities as to cause harm, but there are some herbs which are contra-indicated in pregnancy. Goldenseal should not be used in pregnancy although it may be useful in stimulating and maintaining labour (see below).

Herbs that should NOT be used in pregnancy

Aloe vera	Southernwood
Autumn crocus	Tansy
Barberry	Thuja
Broom	Wormwood
Juniper	Feverfew
Pennyroyal	Sassafras
Poke root	Goldenseal
Parsley	

How to take herbs

There are several different ways of taking herbs depending on whether they are fresh or dried. It is also possible to buy them in liquid form as fluid extracts or tinctures, or as powders which can be used to make into poultices or pastes, or to put into capsules that can be swallowed. Herbs are also made into ointments.

The most common way of using herbs at home to treat pregnancy sickness are by teas, infusions or decoctions. An infusion is made from the aerial parts of a plant, those parts which are above the ground i.e. the leaves, stalks or flowers. It is made by placing either a teaspoonful of the dried herb or three teaspoonsful of the fresh herb into a container such as a teapot and then pouring on a cupful of boiling mineral water. This should be covered and allowed to stand for 15 minutes without further heating. It can then be strained and drunk while still warm.

A decoction is made from the hard, woody parts of a plant – the roots, rhizomes or stems. These need to be boiled to release their properties. Cut, chop or crush the plant as much as possible before putting it into a stainless steel or enamel saucepan. Add cold water using 1 pint (660 ml) to 1 oz (25 g) of dried herb or 3 oz (75 g) of the fresh herb. Bring it to the boil and then let it simmer for 15 minutes or more.

Allow it to infuse off the heat and then strain it and drink it while it is still warm.

Both infusions and decoctions should be used within 24 hours; but they can be kept and reheated to a temperature below boiling. If you find them helpful see if you can get your partner to make up a day's supply each evening so that all you need do next day is warm it up when you need it. Alternatively, you may prefer freezing it in cubes which you can suck. Try combining different herbs to find which are most appealing and effective. Some herb teas are available in tea bags which are convenient for making tea at your bedside if you have a thermos full of hot water. Fennel is available as an instant drink designed for babies. With serious sickness it is probably best to make your own teas, either using fresh herbs or dried ones from a herbalist with a rapid turnover of stock.

Helen Stapleton (1995), a respected midwife-herbalist, recommends drinking the herbs in rotation over a few days as their curative effect may be diminished as you develop a tolerance for them.

Herbs that may be of use in pregnancy sickness

Infusions of:

Chamomile

Peppermint

Hops

Lemon balm

Meadowsweet

Black horehound

Gentian

Raspberry leaf
  (from 14 weeks onwards)

Fennel

Spearmint

Irish moss (Iceland moss is
  often suggested but has not
  been available since the
  Chernobyl disaster)

Ginger (see also p. 71)

Try as a decoction of fresh grated root. Reid (1987) suggests 3–8 g taken as 2–3 drinks during the day, as crystallised stem ginger, in ginger marmalade, biscuits or cakes. You can try it in ginger ale or beer or take the powdered root in capsules available from health food shops and Baldwin's (see p. 119 for details). It can be bought combined with honey in granule form for an instant drink from oriental food shops.

Slippery Elm Bark

This is the powdered bark of the slippery elm tree and a very useful remedy in pregnancy sickness because it is nutritious as well as soothing to the stomach. In herbal terms it is known as a *demulcent*, which means a soothing substance, and its qualities are due to its mucilaginous nature which means that it slips down easily. It is also particularly good at bedtime as it helps you to sleep. There are several ways of taking it; you may need to experiment to find the one that suits you best.

Take a teaspoonful of the powder and mix it with a little cold water to a thin smooth paste. Pour on 1 pint of boiling water or milk while stirring hard. Add sugar to taste, or it can be flavoured with cinnamon, nutmeg or lemon rind.

Slippery Elm Food is available commercially. This is a proprietary product that includes other ingredients such as wheat and oat flour and is described as a sustaining food for infants and invalids.

If you want to take slippery elm without tasting it you can put the powder into 0- or 00-size gelatine capsules and take them several times a day (also available from Baldwin's, see p. 119).

Spicy teas
Some herbalists recommend teas made from spices. You will probably already know if they are likely to suit you – women often find the smell of spices nauseating. American herbalists Vicki Pitman (1994) and Michael Tierra (1980) suggest teas either made of equal parts of cinnamon, cardamom, peppermint or clove or nutmeg. You could also try mixing the following:

3 parts cinnamon
1 part clove
1 part cardamom
1 part nutmeg.

You can either make this with $1/4$–$1/2$ teaspoonful per cup of water, or mix the powders with honey and eat them when you need them.

Ayurvedic medicine from India recognises the value of ginger in treating pregnancy sickness and stomach disorders, as well as for relieving flatulence. It is known as *maha-aushadi* or *vishwabhesaj* – the great medicine or universal healer.

Indian women are expected to display food aversions and cravings when newly pregnant, and are advised to take teas made from fenugreek and coriander seeds. Coriander leaves are regarded as being both stimulant and tonic so that they strengthen the stomach and promote its action. Try eating them fresh, or as a tea, combined with cumin seed – 1 teaspoonful of cumin seed with 1 teaspoonful of chopped coriander leaves to a cup of boiling water. This can be good for sleeplessness and so it is a good tea to take at bedtime.

Chinese women with pregnancy sickness would be likely to try a herbal remedy before resorting to acupuncture. Bob Flaws (1983), an acupuncturist, says he has found the Pinellia and Hoelen combination of herbs (available from Acumedic, see p. 116) very successful in treating pregnancy sickness, especially that deriving from 'Rotten and Muddy *Qi* rebelling upward due to pregnancy'. The symptoms are: intestinal swelling, chest congestion, mental depression and hiccups and belching of 'offensive energy'. (For the differential diagnoses when acupuncture would be better see p. 83.)

If you have access to a peach tree you may like to try making an infusion of its leaves. Jethro Kloss (1985) describes this as a remedy particularly suited to morning sickness and vomiting. The leaves should be picked in July and August and dried for out-of-season use.

· *Homeopathy* ·

Homeopathy is a method of healing that is growing in popularity. It was discovered in 1796 by a German, Samuel Hahnemann. He found that when he gave minute doses of drugs which mimicked the symptoms of an illness to people who actually had the illness, they recovered. For example, taking cinchona bark will give the symptoms of malaria briefly, but taken in a homeopathic dilution it will actually cure it. He described this as 'let like be cured by like' – which is the principle on which homeopathy is based.

The symptoms of illness are regarded by homeopaths as the body's reaction to illness and its attempts to overcome the disease. Homeopathic remedies are designed to strengthen that reaction so that the body can overcome the illness and heal itself.

Because homeopathic dosages are so small they may be safely used for children and pregnant women. If you consult a homeopath, he or she will take a detailed history of your illness, your general state of health, likes and dislikes, what makes you feel better or worse, and get an idea of your temperament and energy level. When the homeopath has a clear picture of you he or she will prescribe a remedy for you that is particularly suited to your needs, so that you might get a different remedy from someone who had similar problems, or you might respond differently to someone given the same remedy as you. Once your homeopath knows you, you may be able to consult by phone.

However, it can be difficult to find the time and energy to see someone new when you are feeling exhausted, and you may be able to treat yourself by matching your pregnancy sickness to the descriptions which follow. Many health food stores and chemists stock a range of homeopathic remedies, usually at the 6C level. For the more unusual remedies, or those at a different strength, you will need to contact a homeopathic pharmacy. There are several which will take your order by phone and their pharmacists are usually very helpful and can give you advice if you want specific information about the remedies. They will usually post your medicine the same day.

You may appreciate how tiny the amount of the active material is in a homeopathic tablet if you know how they are made. The remedies come in different strengths, but unlike pharmaceuticals, the most dilute ones are considered to be the most powerful. There are thousands of remedies all described in a thick bible-like book called the *Materia Medica* (1927). Most are prepared from plant material, although some are made from minerals and things like gold and sand which are generally regarded as inert. They are prepared by serial dilution from a mother tincture which is made from the herb mashed in water. This means that one drop of the tincture is diluted with nine or ninety-nine drops of the diluting medium, depending on whether the potency is to be decimal (X) or centesimal (C). The mixture is shaken vigorously (succussed) and then one drop from that mixture is taken and diluted again in the same ratio. The first dilution becomes 1C or X, the second 2C or X, etc. The potency that is most widely available in shops is 6C (although the C may be missing so that it might appear as *Nux Vomica* 6). The names are often abbreviated too, so that *Antimonium Tartrate* may be known as *Ant.Tart.* for example.

If you would like to try treating your pregnancy sickness homeo-pathically yourself, see which of the following pictures matches your symptoms most closely. You may find it best to get someone else to ask you questions about the way you feel and work it out together. If the one you choose does not seem to help, choose the next nearest, or consult a homeopath (see p. 116–117 for details of how to find one).

Patterns of pregnancy sickness symptoms and the recommended homeopathic treatment (Kaplan, 1994; Ford, 1986)

Actaea racemosa
This is suitable when morning sickness is associated with tension headaches and anxiety. You may be a nervous person who experiences twitching and rheumatic pains affecting the large muscle groups.

Anacardium
Try this if you retch every morning but feel better as soon as you eat

something. You will feel better after eating and if you keep something in your stomach at all times.

Antimonium tartrate
Useful when vomiting occurs immediately you have eaten. It is usually due to undigested food and typically accompanied by collapse and exhaustion. The condition produces a lot of mucus – thick, white or mixed with bile (yellow). The mucus is sometimes stringy, the vomiting is sudden, spasmodic and severe.

Argentum nitricum
This is applicable when considerable flatulence accompanies nausea and vomiting, and you crave sugar and sweet foods. You may feel a panicky nervousness, dislike heat and want cool fresh air.

Cocculus
Try Cocculus if you match any of the following descriptions:

- Travelling by car makes you sick, or you are nauseated by the smell of food.
- You may be averse to food, drink and tobacco.
- You may also have a metallic taste in your mouth.
- You feel over-stressed by disturbed nights, and may be light-haired, sensitive, and romantic.
- Your concentration is poor and you have headaches, abdominal pain as if from sharp stones, and feel dull, lethargic and irritable.
- You also have weakness of the abdominal muscles, and vertigo with a spinning sensation.

Colchicum autumnale
This may help if the smell of food aggravates the problem.

Ipecacuanha
Try this standard remedy for morning sickness if:

- You have constant and persistent nausea and vomiting with excessive salivation.
- There is mucus and bile in your vomit.
- You are irritable but not thirsty.
- You have constant nausea with a clean tongue.
- Vomiting tends to occur after any food.
- Your stomach is irritable and sometimes distended.

Nux vomica
Take this when:

- Vomiting occurs in sudden spasms after breakfast with bitter acid-tasting vomit.

- Your lower stomach feels as if it contains a heavy weight, you have constipation and are very irritable until the afternoon especially if vomiting occurs every morning.
- You are hypersensitive, made angry by stress, sleep badly, have morning sickness and feel as if you have a hangover.
- You have lost your appetite.
- You also have regular or frequent bowel movements but your rectum never feels empty.
- Your tongue is coated and brown.

Petroleum

This may help if, despite persistent nausea and vomiting you never lose your appetite and can eat immediately after vomiting.

Phosphorus

This is of use if you are thirsty for cold water but vomit as soon as it gets warm in your stomach. One dose may be enough.

Pulsatilla

Your symptoms may be variable, e.g:

- You have nausea, cannot tolerate heat or anything fatty or greasy.
- You are not thirsty and only want cold acidic drinks.
- Your tongue has a thick whitish-yellow coating.
- You feel tearful, passive and want sympathy.
- You crave spicy or salty foods, and your abdomen is bloated, rumbling and colicky.

Sepia

This may be of help with the following symptoms:

- You have no lack of appetite despite nausea and vomiting, in fact it may be insatiable.
- Your vomit is pale and contains mucus, and vomiting is followed by exhaustion, fatigue and irritability.
- You are constipated and have low dragging abdominal pains with a general sense of emptiness.
- You frequently feel indifferent, depressed, frustrated, sulky and irritable especially with your family.
- Your skin is sallow with pigmented patches.
- Morning sickness becomes a gnawing hunger only relieved by eating.

Sulphur

Try this if you have burning acid vomit which has an offensive smell and find you are very hungry but eating is followed by vomiting or a sense of weight-like discomfort, often worse on waking: try it also if you have diarrhoea and some skin itching or rash.

Symphoricarpos racemosa
This is indicated when you have persistent vomiting due to pregnancy and nausea from motion and you are averse to all food. Use it when there are no other indications, or if your first remedy fails to work.

Tabacum
This is useful when you have nausea, are pale, chilly and producing excess saliva, while sometimes experiencing continuous, unrelieved nausea without vomiting and have a faint, sinking feeling in your stomach. You feel better in the cold.

To use the remedies

To use a remedy take one tablet, three times a day for two to three days. If your condition is acute you may need to dose yourself more often, perhaps as often as every 15 minutes. When you start to improve, increase the interval between the doses until the improvement is established and then stop. Sometimes the remedy will seem to make the condition worse (known as an aggravation), in which case stop it altogether. This will probably be followed by a big improvement. Only restart the remedy if the symptoms recur. You should generally only take one remedy at a time and avoid other medicines as they may detract from the remedy's efficiency.

The remedies come as tablets or powders, which should be allowed to dissolve under the tongue. Tablets are usually hard and take some time to dissolve but soft, rapidly-dissolving ones are available from Galen's pharmacy by post (see p. 118). They should be taken in a clean mouth, which means that you should not have anything to eat or drink for about 20–30 minutes before or after taking the remedy. You should avoid coffee and peppermint while you are using homeopathy because they may act as antidotes. You may need to buy a special toothpaste designed for users of homeopathy. You should also avoid using the essential oils of Black Pepper, Camphor, Eucalyptus or the Mints as they may also prevent the remedies from working.

The medicines are sensitive and can easily become contaminated so they should be stored in a cool, dark place well away from strong smells. Keep them in their original containers and tip the pills out into the lid when you want to take one so that you do not touch any that need to be put back. The remedies can also be taken in warm water; this is particularly suitable for acute conditions where doses need to be taken frequently. Crush two tablets and dissolve them in warm water and sip it slowly.

· *Aromatherapy* ·

Like most other alternative medical therapies, the use of essential oil and unguents goes back to earliest times. Oils and unguents were used in rituals for religious purposes and therapeutically for treating illness, as well as in cooking. Vedic literature from India listed over 700 substances more than 2000 years BC and the Chinese include aromatics within details of their ancient herbal tradition recorded in *The Yellow Emperor's Book of Internal Medicine* written at around the same time. An Egyptian papyrus records the use of medicinal herbs some 800 years before that, while about 2000 BC the Egyptians were renowned for their use of oils and unguents, some of which, like cedar and myrrh, were used in the embalming processes. Traces of the oils they used are detected by archaeologists today.

However, despite the widespread use of plants and spices in healing throughout many centuries, aromatherapy, which is now becoming well known, was only rediscovered in 1928, by a French chemist, Gattefosse. He was working in his family's perfume business and accidentally discovered the healing properties of the essential oil of lavender when he burnt his arm severely and plunged it into the oil, to find that it healed without scarring.

Essential oils work in three ways: pharmacologically, physiologically and psychologically. An essential oil can effect chemical changes within the body and reacts with hormones and enzymes. It acts physiologically by bringing about changes within the body – stimulating, sedating etc. Its psychological effect occurs when a person reacts to its smell.

Various combinations of oils are described as refreshing, uplifting, soothing, harmonising, sensual, detoxifying or good for aches or pains. There is a good combination for use in labour which relieves pain and tension, containing rose, jasmine, geranium, clary sage and lavender. It should only be used at the end of pregnancy because of a theoretical risk of stimulating premature contractions if used earlier.

Not all plants yield the essential oils, which are regarded as their life-blood and defence against disease, and some yield much more than others, which partly reflects the disparity in price. Much more information about essential oils can be obtained from Julia Lawless's excellent *Encyclopaedia of Essential Oils* (Lawless, 1992).

The oils are prepared by a process of distillation, or pressure applied to oils such as that from citrus fruits. Distillation is achieved by steam, water or solvent distillation.

Essential oils may be used in pregnancy although at half the dose normally prescribed for adults and with the proviso that some oils are not used at all and some not in the first 14 weeks (see below). Some oils are the subject of debate: they appear to have been used safely by pregnant women in the past (and are recommended by some experienced aromatherapists) but some, such as lavender and peppermint, have constituents which theoretically may be *emmenagogues,* i.e. encourage the menstrual cycle, and in pregnancy are regarded as abortifacients. These are not recommended in the first trimester (up to 14 weeks) or at all if you have any reason to consider your pregnancy at risk, e.g. if you have had bleeding in this pregnancy or have a history of miscarriage. There are a number of different ways of using essential oils: choose the way that seems most appropriate or convenient. When buying essential oils, make sure that they are 100% pure oil as some that are widely available are diluted (see p. 116 for details of a reliable supplier).

How to use aromatherapy oils

The following four methods describe how you can use aromatherapy but you *must* remember to **halve these dosages in pregnancy.**

Bath
Make a 6% blend by adding 6 drops of essential oil to 5 ml teaspoon of base which can be either full cream milk or vodka. This disperses the oil, which may otherwise sting or irritate. If your bath is acrylic or fibreglass, you should wipe the oil off the bath afterwards.

Massage oil
7–25 drops to 25 ml base oil
3–5 drops to a 5 ml tsp base oil
20–60 drops to 100 ml base oil
Use oil such as sweet almond or grapeseed as a base and get someone to massage them in. This will feel pleasant and ensure they are absorbed into the bloodstream, but you can massage them in to any accessible part of your body yourself equally as effectively.

Hot and cold compresses
Add a few drops of essential oil to a bowl of very hot or ice cold water. Dip in a flannel or piece of cotton, squeeze it out and apply it to the affected area, allow it to cool (or warm) and repeat. For pregnancy sickness try hot compresses over the abdomen. These are also useful for

backaches, toothaches, etc, when hot, or headaches, sprains, etc, when cold.

Vaporisation

You can put a few drops of oil into a bowl of warm water and place it on a radiator, or you can buy a special burner or a metal ring that can be placed over a light bulb to warm a few drops. Alternatively, you can add a drop to a corner of your pillow or on a handkerchief to smell during the day. Smelling essential oils in this way is quite safe; any smell which you find helpful in relieving nausea may be used.

There are other methods of using essential oils such as steam inhalation, skin oils and lotions and douches, but none are applicable to pregnancy sickness. The oils should not be used neat on the skin or taken internally.

Essential oils useful in alleviating pregnancy sickness

You will be aware of any that smell disagreeable to you while you are pregnant.

Suitable for use in a massage oil

Ginger	Petitgrain
Grapefruit	Sweet orange
Lime	Tangerine
Mandarin	

Added to a bowl of water by your bed or put on a corner of your pillow

Petitgrain	Lemon
Roman chamomile	Spearmint
Coriander	Peppermint
Lavender (*Lavendula angustifolia*)	

The following oils are contra-indicated but it is still safe to take infusions of some of the herbs that are listed, e.g. fennel, clove.

Essential oils to be avoided in pregnancy

Ajowan	Boldo
Aniseed	Buchu
Basil	Camphor
Birch	Clove
Bitter Almond	Cornmint

Fennel
Horseradish
Hyssop
Lavender cotton
Lavendula stoechas
Mugwort
Mustard
Myrrh
Oregano
Parsleyseed
Pennyroyal
Pimenta racemosa
Plecanthrus

Rue
Salvia officinalis
Savin
Savory
Star Aniseed
Tansy
Tarragon
Thuja
Thyme (thymol type)
Wintergreen
Wormseed
Wormwood

· *Hypnotherapy* ·

Hypnotherapy has a place in treating pregnancy sickness not only because its exponents claim it works, but because it is drug-free and once learned can be practised at home, with the additional benefit that it may be used for relieving pain during labour.

Hypnosis works in several ways but it is important to appreciate that you are neither asleep nor unconscious while being hypnotised and that the hypnotherapist is not able to control your mind or behaviour against your will. You may only be hypnotised if you agree to it, and want and expect it to work. A hypnotherapist will help you reach a state of deep relaxation and enable you to concentrate intensely on a limited area of attention. You will find that you have a heightened level of responsiveness to suggestions or cues or signals made by the therapist. Your critical faculty will be reduced so that it will be as if you have no past experience of the subject and thus able to take suggestions at face value.

A hypnotherapist treating pregnancy sickness might suggest that you are particularly sensitive to pregnancy hormones such as oestrogen and human chorionic gonadotrophin, and that it is possible for you to reset your nausea centre like resetting a thermostat. As it is turned down you will become less sensitive to the hormones and gain control of your symptoms.

Baram (1995) states that 80% of women with severe morning sickness will improve following hypnosis, some after only one treatment – even those so severely ill that they are unable to swallow their own saliva.

Another effect of hypnotherapy includes the opportunity to explore unpleasant feelings associated with past experiences. One practitioner (Arthurs, 1994) believes that nausea and vomiting in pregnancy and *hyperemesis gravidarum* are symptoms of emotional rather than physical distress, caused by a traumatic emotion which has been suppressed and shows itself as emesis. Under hypnosis it is possible to explore your relationships with the baby's father, your other children and family and your partner's family, and the effect pregnancy may have on your career and relationship with your partner. He believes that if you can explore any ambivalence about the pregnancy and concern you have about the health of the baby, and other stresses and conflicts in your life, it will result in improvement of pregnancy sickness symptoms.

Henker (1970) described treating women with intractable (nothing-can-help) nausea and vomiting in pregnancy with hypnotic suggestion, behaviour therapy and supportive psychotherapy, and found that within two days they were better than women in the control group, although not all the controls were in hospital. Another team of researchers (Apfel, Kelly & Frankel, 1986) considered that in fact women with the more severe form of sickness, *hyperemesis gravidarum*, were treated more successfully with hypnosis than those with milder symptoms.

At the end of treatment a hypnotherapist will encourage you to come out of your deep relaxation and perhaps give you a tape so that you will be able to listen to it and practise the technique of self-hypnosis at home. You may be taught a technique that you can practise at any time to reduce nausea. There is no risk of becoming stuck in a trance, and you should find that you are able to make desirable changes in your habits and that your motivation and self-image are generally improved. If you have hypnotherapy in order to treat pregnancy sickness you will know very soon if it is effective.

· *Maria O'Brien* ·

I was nauseous with my first pregnancy but only sick a couple of times and the nausea stopped at around 13–14 weeks. This time I found out I was pregnant at about five weeks and at the same time I started to feel sick. Initially I felt nauseous in the morning but by the time I was 9–10 weeks pregnant it was lasting all through the day. My husband was away on a school skiing trip, when it was at its peak.

I was being sick at least every other day: sometimes I would eat and be sick almost immediately, before the food was digested. I also felt faint – I never did faint but I was worried that I would when I was on my own at home with Eoin. He was only fourteen months and didn't know what was happening when I was sick. I felt helpless, being sick with him hanging on to my leg, and I felt I had to try and do my best and get over it for his sake.

At the time I was working with a class of 8–9 year olds. Fortunately I was part-time and so able to do only two or three days a week, my school was understanding about that. I explained to my class that I was pregnant and what was involved and they were very good about it. They appreciated that when it was PE I might have to sit on the side instead of joining in. They seemed to realise when I was feeling particularly bad, and be nicer.

The mother of one child in my class was expecting her fifth child at around the same time and her daughter was especially understanding; she used to notice how I looked and would ask how I felt. However, I did have to rush out of class a few times, telling a teacher in one of the other rooms that I was going. It's better being sick in the comfort of your own home – I found it embarrassing being sick when there were other people in the toilet listening to me.

I found, too, that I had to be careful. If I wolfed my dinner down, perhaps because there were clubs after lunch, it would come straight up again. Initially I thought I was suffering from a bug because it was so different from my first experience of pregnancy.

I used to find that fizzy drinks helped, especially Lucozade or those with ginger in. I kept a bottle of still Lucozade in my desk drawer and used to line drinks up in front of me on my desk and work my way through them sipping them little and often. It didn't matter that a bottle was already open because it was flat to start with. I also ate a lot of Clarnico mints with peppermint oil in them – they seemed to help. I felt worst when I hadn't eaten and I found ginger biscuits helped. There are some old-fashioned cookies made by Tesco's that have got pieces of stem ginger in them that are really strong and those were very good. I used to keep some by my bedside and have one first thing in the morning with a mouthful during the night sometimes. I kept squash or lemon barley water there too. I was lucky that my husband had time to bring me a morning cup of chamomile tea while I was still in bed.

The other thing that really helped was my Sea-bands. I don't know how much of it was in my mind but I really didn't dare take them off in the shower or even to wash them – they got really grubby. I lent them to a friend while I was not pregnant and she felt exactly the same way about them .

Some things made it worse. The doctor gave me magnesium trisilicate but I tried it once and was sick immediately so I didn't bother again. I'm sure being tired and rundown made it worse too. I found it the worst kind of illness – much worse than anything else.

My nausea and vomiting suddenly stopped, literally overnight, at 18 weeks. I just woke up one morning and I felt fine – it was wonderful. However, I had felt ill for nearly half the pregnancy and I had said to my husband if ever I want another child just remind me of how awful I'm feeling now. I wonder about that; I've always wanted a large family, but what if it was worse? My friend has just had a third baby and says she got worse each time. Someone in my antenatal class was sick until 33 weeks. I want to enjoy pregnancy, not resent it. And yet other people have no symptoms – I really envy them.

Maria subsequently had Aidan, a 6lb 5oz boy.

Chapter Eleven

HOW YOUR SICKNESS AFFECTS THOSE AROUND YOU

You're feeling rotten and exhausted as well, but is everyone going to rally round and help you out? With luck they will, but there are a variety of reasons why you may not get the support that you feel you deserve.

· *Your partner* ·

Although he may be sympathetic, it can be very difficult for people to really understand the impact that pregnancy sickness has on someone if they haven't had it themselves. It is very hard to imagine feeling that ill day after day and, moreover, sympathy does run out eventually. It can be compared with colic in babies, which lasts on average for the same length of time. At first you feel desperately sorry for the baby, but as time wears on and nothing that you do appears to make any difference, you start to lose patience. The fact that your tiny baby is in evident pain no longer affects you in the same way and you may begin to feel resentful and in need of sympathy yourself. Of course in neither case can a baby or a woman be blamed for their symptoms, nor has anything improved, but the capacity for sympathy in others has diminished.

Pregnancy sickness can have an isolating effect on men too. They may find, as some have said, that they find themselves leading separate lives, cooking for themselves and eating alone. They are thrust into a caring role several months before they expected to be, and may find it hard to accept a change of lifestyle that means their social life is restricted. They are having to cope and cook, their wife or partner is nothing like the person she used to be, she is changing, her interests have altered, and life is not as much fun as it was before she became pregnant. Discussion may be out of the question with someone who either has her head down the loo – or is passionate about going to bed – to sleep.

Besides which sickness cannot in any sense be described as a glamorous illness. Its smell and sounds are distinctly off-putting. However, your partner is invaluable because he can:

- read the book with/for you
- organise and prepare remedies
- get or buy things to help
- make appointments
- sort out changes to your lifestyle
- arrange extra sleep
- talk about it

He is also in a good position to make an objective assessment about whether you are too ill to work or so dehydrated that you need to be admitted to hospital.

· *Keith Wilson* ·
(husband of Caroline – see p. 77)

I always felt very sorry for her, I know how ghastly being sick is. I felt sorry that it made her so weak as well.

With the first pregnancy it didn't really inconvenience me but I well remember the time we were driving to Oban in Scotland and she was sick for the first time before we left Ealing. It didn't augur well and she was sick loads of times before we got there.

It's a dim and distant memory now and I look at our healthy children and thank God for them and think it's worth going through it for them.

· *Paul Stark* ·
(husband of Liliana – see p. 42)

I remember it as being most severe when Lili was expecting Ben and Kylie was three. Lili was in three different hospitals for a period totalling three and a half months. The last one she was in was the other side of London and through horrendous traffic. I used to have to get Kylie up at 6.30am, clothe and feed her and drag her off to the childminder to be there at 7.30am. Kylie wasn't happy there – although the childminder was a lovely person. She used to tell me that Kylie would grieve all day, not just when I left her. I often used to leave her there in tears myself.

I'd pick her up at 6.00pm and we would spend an hour and a half driving to see Lili who often wasn't well enough to be seen. If she was we would spend a quarter of an hour with her and drive back to be home by 9.30pm. I'd get Kylie undressed and ready for bed, cook for myself and get ready for the next day.

My parents helped at the weekend but they were both working and my mother wasn't well either. It was traumatic – although the baby was growing, Lili kept on losing weight. I didn't feel we had much support from the medical profession; they tended to dismiss us, saying Lili was imagining it.

I try NOT to remember, it was so traumatic. Kylie became more unhappy as time went by. She was alright with me and I tried to work from home more, take time off and even took her with me. I'm a building site surveyor, but it was no fun at all.

· *Your children* ·

Unless they are much older, children are unlikely to be able to make fewer demands because you don't feel well. Young children often resent their mother feeling ill, because they expect a mother to be fit, capable and in control, with the strength and energy to care for them. They may be able to be sympathetic briefly, but then they will carry on as normal, or become more demanding because they sense their world as being less stable.

You may not want to explain to your children just yet why you feel ill; it can be hard to fend off questions about whether the baby will be born today when you are in the early months of pregnancy, and young children find it difficult to deal with a long wait.

And if you do tell your children you have to be prepared for the world, including the plumber, to know all about it!

· *Your mother* ·

Surely your mother will be sympathetic – after all, she has been pregnant at least once. But not necessarily, as the stories show. Certainly some women describe wonderful mothers who have moved in and taken over or who have had their daughters and their existing children to stay, but others have not found it so easy to be understanding. Quite a few women with pregnancy sickness have said that because their mothers had not experienced it themselves they tended to feel that their daughters were exaggerating the extent of their illness or really only needed to pull themselves together. Although in some ways, in the past, pregnancy was accorded more respect, other prevailing attitudes encouraged women not to complain and to 'get on with' what was considered to be 'a woman's lot'.

Grandmothers and grandmothers-to-be are often working outside their homes nowadays and may find it difficult to get time off to help you in the way that you would like. Some may not relish the change of role or category that becoming a granny implies or feel envious of your pregnancy.

· *Friends* ·

Your friends may be your best bet, especially if they have been pregnant and suffered similarly recently. Many women find that a subsequent pregnancy does not rate as much attention amongst their family as the first, but they have the advantage of having made friends with women who were pregnant at the time they were expecting their first babies, with whom they share a common bond, and who may well be pregnant at around the same time in their subsequent pregnancies. Talking to other sufferers can be very helpful indeed and it can be wonderful if someone with a child of similar age to yours will give you some spare time to sleep. Caroline Wilson and Caroline Davis (see pp. 25 and 77) both severe sufferers and friends, were pregnant and sick alternately so that they were able to support each other through it.

However, friends who have not been pregnant or those who have sailed blithely through pregnancy may not realise how you feel and you may have to ask for help directly rather than trusting to their intuition. Most people are good at assisting when they know that they are wanted and needed.

All of which may sound negative, but hopefully you will find that giving this book to your helpers so that they can read about other people's experience of pregnancy sickness will help them to realise how it is affecting you. The suggestions for how to improve the situation should give them something that they can do, and reduce their feeling of helplessness. (For Kirsten's account see p. 47.)

· *Mark Elliott* ·

I felt guilty that I wasn't there when Kirsten had the threatened miscarriage. I'd just started a new job and was keen to impress, so I was at a function in London. I got back late and crept in quietly so as not to wake Kirsten. I undressed in the dark and went into the bedroom and found she wasn't there. Then the hospital rang to say 'we've got your partner here'. I went on feeling guilty about the fact that there was such difficulty in curing the sickness, and that I wasn't around to help. I did rush 85 miles home quickly three days a week and I worked in London and from home as much as possible.

We had recently spent four years living in Scotland so we were new to the area and had few friends around. I hated having to leave Kirsten here during the day, on her own and ill.

I think there was a lack of professional support on a regular basis. She'd be treated while she was in hospital but as soon as we were out of their hair it was forgotten. It was a bit like a pit stop for Damon Hill: they would attend to the situation when it was in front of them but as soon as she was rehydrated she was out again. When the routine drug solutions failed to work – and they tried everything from Dioralyte and oral treatments to suppositories – they just seemed to consider there was no answer. No one talked about any alternative methods of treatment like homeopathy. They just offered things like a sip of water or a suppository, and when it wasn't successful they just said it would all be over by February.

There was good backup – from the midwives and health visitor after Flora was born. But it would have been nice to have had that during the particular problems of the pregnancy.

It would also have been good to review the situation after the birth to discuss what had happened and look at the future. I think we should have been referred to someone who was a specialist in this condition who would tell us about it and what could be done to ameliorate it.

· *Michael* ·

Imagine trying to have a relationship with someone who has their head in a bucket or a bowl constantly. The man has to do everything! I would come home from work and have to take over the lot: cooking, laundry and looking after Calum. As soon as I got in, Alison went to bed.

We had buckets and towels everywhere and it was my job to go around looking in them to see if they needed slopping out – there was never very much in them though. Not surprisingly, it made Alison very irritable; she was noticeably short-tempered.

Although it sounds unsympathetic, it's not much fun listening to someone retching all the time. In fact morning sickness doesn't warrant much sympathy. People think it is natural and that you've brought it on yourself. Because it is not life-threatening and you know it will end eventually, it's not taken very seriously.

· *Work* ·

People's work situations are too varied to make recommendations about, and you will know yourself how time off for sickness is regarded by your employer.

Although it is illegal for women to be sacked or discriminated against merely for being pregnant, it is quite clear that pregnancy is often not welcomed by employers and possibly it will result in your being passed over for promotion or be held against you in some other way. Although women should not be discriminated against for being pregnant, it still happens and pregnancy sickness may cause particular difficulties for people who work for small employers, or those who are free-lance or self-employed, for whom time off work means no pay.

Maternity Alliance – an organisation concerned with the rights of and services for mothers, fathers and babies – says that many women do try to conceal pregnancy symptoms as employers can be resentful of the trouble pregnancy may cause them.

Legally, a person may not be discriminated against for any reason to do with pregnancy. Moreover, any time off related to sickness as a result of pregnancy must be recorded separately from that caused by general sickness so that it may not be included in a person's sickness record, if for example redundancy is being considered.

However Maternity Alliance is aware that many women are victimised as a result of their pregnancies, and there is little redress unless it is so severe as to force them to leave their jobs which they are reluctant to do when expecting a baby.

Women evidently are good at overcoming or concealing the difficulties that pregnancy sickness can cause – few of the personnel officers that I spoke to, including several directors of midwifery who might have been expected to be particularly aware of problems caused by pregnancy, considered it a problem, apart from those women who were admitted to hospital with *hyperemesis gravidarum*.

The legislation regarding maternity rights is changing all the time. For up-to-date information you can get a leaflet 'Pregnant at Work' by sending an SAE together with a first-class stamp to cover costs to:

Maternity Alliance
45 Beech St
London EC2P 2LX
Tel: 0171 588 8582

If you feel able to reveal your pregnancy you will at least be in a stronger position to take time off if you are too ill to work. If however, you still want to keep it quiet, you can either cope by trying the suggestions in the book, especially zinc, or get a sickness certificate from your doctor with a non-specific description of your illness.

Obviously there are all sorts of reasons for wanting to keep it quiet, but commonly there is a desire not to tell anyone before the pregnancy is felt to be secure. This is fine if you are able to do it and it can be fun to keep the secret to yourselves for a while – but it can also be fun to share it. It is worth knowing that parents who lose babies before anyone knows that they are expected often regret not having told people about the baby in the early weeks of pregnancy. Miscarriage occurs more often than many women appreciate, and the point made by bereaved parents is that if no one knows you were pregnant no one will acknowledge your loss, which will be a very real one. Waiting until you are past the customary 13–14 weeks can only be lovely if you continue to be pregnant or are not so ill that it becomes a strain.

If you want to keep your pregnancy quiet because of its effect on your future employment your partner may be able to help to come to a decision about how ill you really are and how serious the threat to your job is. Bear in mind that motherhood does change things, and while your job may be of great importance to you at the moment, you may feel differently once your baby is born. (You may not believe me but it is true.)

Provided pregnancy goes well you will have to tell your employer at some point, and if you are feeling really ill it might as well be sooner as later. Larger companies may have the capacity to cope with staff illness and be able to provide extra rest or ease your workload. You may want to be independent and cope alone, but the opportunity for your employers to help the next generation is there if it gets too difficult. In other jobs it may be hard to get time off, or to rest during the day. Teachers, for example, can find it difficult even to find the time to be sick when they are at work. One teacher told of working in a classroom hut without easy access to a lavatory where she had to keep a bucket in a cupboard in which to be sick.

It may help you to consider the following questions:

- If this illness was caused by anything other than pregnancy, e.g. a virus, would I take time off?
- Am I coping, or seeming to cope?
- Am I being silly? Should I really be in bed?

Of course there are advantages in being at work: many of the severe sufferers who tell their stories say that being at work was better than being at home, because it took their minds off their sickness and prevented them from giving in to it; some said it helped to be in an environment where there was no kitchen.

You may feel guilty about the effect your pregnancy has on your colleagues' work-load, but as has also been remarked, 'Motherhood is guilt.' Perhaps if you can be open about your illness without making too much of it, you will find your colleagues are helpful and happy for you.

· *Clare Pickard* ·

In my pregnancy last time I was sick right through. I conceived in August and was being sick by the beginning of September. To start with I was sick in the mornings and then by the end of October everything turned around and I started feeling queasy at 3 pm and being sick in the evenings. It went on throughout the whole pregnancy, it was very unusual for me to have two consecutive days without being sick; only once was it three.

I did feel better for two weeks at around seven-and-a-half months and then the sickness returned, linked to indigestion. I'd get heartburn and that would bring it on. I think it still would now I am pregnant again, but now I can control it with Rapeze which states it is safe for pregnant women. Last time there was nothing like that, everything said 'not to be taken in pregnancy'. I did try magnesium trisilicate that the doctor gave me but it was too strong and I was sick straightaway.

I stayed at work until a week before Rhiannon was born, 10 days early weighing 6lb 12oz. Being at work helped to cope with feeling ill. I would have been very lonely and depressed at home. I didn't know anyone and it wasn't a sociable time; we only managed to go out once, on my birthday.

My job takes me all over the country and I used to be sick on trains. I could manage the local trains but on Inter-City those huge bends are awful.

My abiding memory of that pregnancy is of being sick and just eating very plain chicken or fish, and carrots which was about all I could manage, although some very plain vegetables like boiled courgettes were possible. Sometimes I had completely plain pasta, never anything with a sauce. I couldn't eat any dairy produce, nor anything with the slightest hint of fat. Very occasionally I could manage an omelette made with almost no fat at all and certainly nothing like cheese in it. I could manage biscuits such as ginger, rich tea – all the ones people suggest – but I couldn't manage anything very sweet which was quite a change for me, and I couldn't manage cereal so I often ended up eating very little.

I did find peppermint tea helped: it helped me to digest my food. Hot lemon barley water made quite weak helped too – it meant I would replace some of the energy lost quite quickly. I had to eat in hotels a lot because of my job as a trainer, and I found the chefs really helpful.

It took me a whole year to feel really well again after my first pregnancy and I couldn't face the thought of pregnancy for quite a while. I thought I might be pregnant at one point and I was horrified. Luckily though, when I conceived again in January, I was only sick until the beginning of March; this pregnancy has been completely different.

Clare has since had a son, Jackson, who weighed 8lb 13oz.

· *Sue Parfitt* ·

I only had a couple of weeks' sickness when I was pregnant with Ben but the second time it started at 8 weeks and went on until 18. Although it doesn't seem long now, at the time it seemed to last forever. They say it stops at 16 weeks and you pin your hopes on that. It's awful when it continues because you have no idea when it will end, and if you already have children you can't give up completely.

I felt sick and I was sick. I used to travel to work with a bucket in the car. At first I didn't want to tell them at work that I was pregnant, but when I did they were reasonably sympathetic provided I was ill in my own time. I did once take a morning off work because I just couldn't manage to go in, otherwise I used to have to rush out of lessons to be sick. I teach home economics which was particularly difficult because I couldn't bear the sight of meat or the smell of it cooking. I had to steer clear of it and teach my pupils to cook things like cakes and biscuits. I remember dashing out once and when I got back one of the children asked, 'Have you been crying, Miss?'

People think of it as you being sick once and then that is it – they don't imagine your being sick over and over again. I always had that weak feeling which was worse when I was tired, but it was useful to have the distraction of working – you just can't give in.

I tried Sea-Bands but they didn't help at all.

It is worrying when you read the pregnancy books and they say how vital it is for the baby to be getting various nutrients while it is developing and you can't keep it down and are losing weight.

I remember cancelling dinner invitations – either I couldn't cook or I couldn't face going out. I think your partner does tend to get fed up with you being a wet blanket all the time.

I was convinced Thomas was going to be a girl because the sickness was so different from the first time and it is supposed to be worse with girls.

· *Christine Asbury* ·

I have had five pregnancies and was sick with all except the one that was ectopic. That includes the baby that I miscarried at 15 weeks, which died in utero when I felt just as sick although it tailed off in the last 2–3 weeks. With my first pregnancy, I felt better by 22 weeks, but with the others I was sick all the way through. It seemed to get worse each time. The first time it happened it was like a bolt from the blue because I wasn't expecting it. It started at six weeks. One morning I felt sick for a few minutes and then it wore off. Two days later I was flat on my back throwing up every few minutes. After two to three weeks of being really ill, I managed to get back to eating again, although I was still sick. I became very dehydrated and lost half a stone, although no one took much interest or suggested I was hospitalised.

I had a week off work but then felt that I couldn't take any longer, so I would sit up, get up and throw up, then struggle into work. Eventually I got it under control so that I could tell when I was going to be sick and manage to get to a loo. I've been sick in various loos, including one of the staff loos in the building society.

With the second, it crept up a bit more slowly: it started earlier but I was expecting it. This time I took Avomine *once I was 12 weeks pregnant. That controlled it quite well although I still felt sickish.*

I found smells very bad. I couldn't go anywhere near the kitchen. If I came back from work and my au pair had cooked fish fingers for the children, I found the smell lingered and I really hated it. I preferred going to work because home smells were worse, especially those of cooking.

I got the trick of carrying air sick bags with me. However, I was once stuck in a queue of traffic and was sick all over my coat. Once I was in control, I could manage not to be sick during the day but I still had a horrible feeling of sickness all day long.

With the third and fourth pregnancies, I thought that I was not going to get it – every pregnancy is different and I thought maybe it won't happen this time. I was particularly hopeful because with both of them I felt really well for the week before the sickness started. Then I was hit by sudden desolation when it started again. With these two, I developed an even more unpleasant symptom, whereby I was sick the instant I had eaten, so that it would return to the plate. With the fourth, I started taking Stemetil *at six weeks, which didn't help at all. Eventually, I was put on to an antihistamine similar to* Avomine, *which made it tolerable although it did no more than take the edge off it.*

I did try all sorts of alternative therapies: homeopathy, acupuncture, herbalism, but none worked in the slightest. I used to go and see a good homeopath who would say cheerfully, 'I think we're getting there,' but after six weeks with no improvement, I didn't think we were. If you go on seeing people for long enough, there's likely to be a natural improvement anyway. My sister went to see an acupuncturist in the Midlands, who said she had a good record of curing pregnancy sickness, but it didn't really make any difference to her either. She is pregnant now with her second child and has been badly affected too, although I don't think she is as sick as me. So far it seems as if it's the boys who make pregnancy sickness worse. My sister is a teacher and has had to have more time off than me because it is a job where you just can't put your head down for five minutes, you are on show all the time. [She gave birth to a girl.]

Our mother is very unsympathetic. She was sick while pregnant too, but feels that you should just cope, although I think she was surprised at how ill I was. It is hard to believe how little sympathy it attracts: people seem to feel that it is all in the mind and that you just need to pull yourself together. I became very irritated by the constant advice to eat a dry cracker, and by those who said, 'I never had that.'

My partner was very supportive, particularly with the first, but he got irritated in the end. He found it very frustrating to have to be both sympathetic and do everything including looking after the children. I would sometimes say that I couldn't bear it and I would swap if I could, but he felt he was worst off. It's probably because you can't imagine unrelenting nausea and it is impossible to describe or convey.

The only things that did help were, at one time, drinking Bovril, and when I went to stay with my mother. I found that not having to decide what to eat or cook, made it easier to keep things down. I've heard that that is what makes things easier if you are admitted to hospital with it; all the decisions are taken away from you. Though people who have been admitted say that it improves while you are there but gets worse once you are back.

I'm sure there is a psychological element which perhaps makes it easier for alternative therapies to work. I found with the first that I felt sick as soon as I had done a positive pregnancy test, although I think it was coincidence, because I knew I was pregnant anyway. I never needed to do another one.

With my fourth pregnancy I had a toddler who was little more than a baby and it was appallingly difficult. Even when feeding him stuff out of jars, I would give him three spoonfuls and then have to rush to the sink to throw up.

Looking back, I think that surely it can't have been that bad but it was. I remember the really bad nausea and that trembly state before throwing up.

My sickness decimated the family, it put me out of action completely for at least two weeks and I could have little to do with food after that, which is why I have decided not to have another child. I feel I couldn't impose that on the family again.

· Head teacher ·

I feel sympathetic about morning sickness because I had it badly myself when I was pregnant twenty or more years ago. I think it was easier then because I taught older children and teaching them was more formal so that I could set them something to do and watch them do it while facing the door. I just managed – as you do.

I have a member of staff who is suffering at the moment. She isn't actually sick but feels it. I keep a careful eye on her and help her with the work-load. If she looks pale, she's obviously not feeling very well and I help her out. However, she didn't want the rest of the staff to know, although she told me she was pregnant as soon as she knew. I had to say that it was important to tell them or they would wonder why she was getting so much help and resent it. I didn't want them complaining. Teaching can be very stressful, especially when you are teaching young children and I always make sure there is someone in with her and make things easier when possible.

Chapter Twelve

YOUR NEXT PREGNANCY

Planning another pregnancy or being pregnant again can cause considerable anxiety if things did not go well last time. If pregnancy sickness was anything more than a minor problem, or if it lasted longer than average, you are bound to wonder whether you would feel the same again or if there is anything that you could do prior to pregnancy that would help to prevent it.

Unfortunately there is some evidence to suggest that if you've had it once you are likely to get it again. However there are plenty of women – some of whom have described the way they were affected in this book – who have felt very ill during one pregnancy and had hardly any symptoms in the next pregnancy. It can work the other way round, of course – which adds to the mystery regarding its cause and ways of preventing it. The good news is that, in general, symptoms are less common in women who are older and those who have already had a full term pregnancy. It is thought that oestrogen production and metabolism are altered by a woman's first full-term pregnancy so that the amount of free oestriol is lower in subsequent pregnancies.

Mothers who already have a child often have a better support network and are in contact with other women going through pregnancy at around the same time. This can be enormously helpful. It's recognised that being able to discuss the problem with a friend or partner is one of the best ways of helping pregnancy sickness. Of course feeling ill while looking after a small child, when it can be impossible to rest, can make you feel much worse. Children are often unable to empathise with their mothers' feeling ill and it may only increase the demands they make.

· Can it be prevented? ·

There are measures you can take and although none are guaranteed to work they are worth trying. Some steps are advisable for anyone planning pregnancy. These include taking a vitamin supplement, particularly one including zinc and folic acid. Taking a multivitamin prior to conception has been shown to reduce fetal abnormalities and also to reduce symptoms of nausea, vomiting and vertigo in pregnancy (see also p. 73 for details of dosages and advice about taking vitamin supplements). Zinc may be especially useful.

If you smoke you should stop, not because it will reduce morning sickness – smokers appear to suffer less – but because smoking increases by 33% the chance of your baby being stillborn or dying at around the time of birth. He or she may suffer oxygen deprivation at birth, be a lower birthweight with consequent long-term health risks and be at increased risk of cot death (Meyer *et al.*, 1976). You can get help in giving up from the Smoker's Quitline – 0800 002200.

If you are overweight you may like to lose some before pregnancy. Some studies show nausea and vomiting in pregnancy is more common in heavier women. It may also be helpful to reduce caffeine from coffee, tea and colas, if you drink a lot of them, particularly if you have problems in conceiving. Some experts feel that caffeine levels and pregnancy sickness are correlated, others that high levels of caffeine reduce the chances of conception.

Although there is no evidence of cause and effect, communities where they eat a lot of green vegetables and whose staple diet is based on maize do not appear to suffer nausea and vomiting in pregnancy. They also eat a diet high in fats. Of course there may also be a genetic component and increasing these in your diet may not reduce the likelihood of having pregnancy sickness. But with the exception of the fats a comparable diet based on food like spinach and polenta can't hurt (Minturn & Weiher, 1984).

If you were so ill last time that you are really doubtful about even having another baby, you will probably want to line up your defences beforehand. Your doctor should be able to refer you to a specialist who will be able to discuss your past pregnancy and future ones with particular reference to the problems you had. He or she should be able to formulate a plan for future treatment should it be needed, and let you know if there's any new treatment that may help you.

It can also be helpful to consult an alternative medical practitioner – whichever therapy appeals to you. Ring round to find someone who has had experience of dealing with and is sympathetic to your difficulties. Most therapists like to have the opportunity to get women into perfect health with no underlying deficiencies at the start of pregnancy, and it could be that starting off that way would minimise any chance of a recurrence. Homeopaths in particular feel that they may be able to treat miasms or underlying family weaknesses that might result in nausea and vomiting in pregnancy.

Good luck!

USEFUL ADDRESSES

Acupuncture

The Acupuncture Association and Register 34 Alderney Street, London SW1. Tel: 0171 834 1012. They will supply a register of acupuncturists and a handbook in return for £2.50.

Acumedic Centre East Asia Co. Ltd 103 Camden High Street, London NW1. Tel: 0171 388 5783. Shop selling books about acupuncture, moxa, needles, etc. Clinic, 9.30–5.30, six days a week, by appointment only.

Aromatherapy

Bach flower remedies
Dr Edward Bach Centre Mount Vernon, Wallingford, Oxon OX10 0PZ. Tel: 01491 839489. Supplies a booklet, *The Twelve Healers*, for 50p.

Chiropractice

British Chiropractic Association 29 Whitley Street, Reading RG2 0EG. Tel: 01734 757557. Will supply a list of qualified chiropracters if you send an SAE and £1.

Complementary medicine

Council for Complementary and Alternative Medicine – Tel: 0171 724 9103. For information send SAE and £1.50 to: 179 Gloucester Place, London NW1 6DX.

Institute of Complementary Medicine Unit 4, Tavern Quay, London SE16 1AA. Tel: 0171 237 5165. For a list of practitioners, send SAE plus two first-class stamps to: PO Box 194, London SE16 1QZ.

Cranial Therapy

Sutherland Cranial College Morecambe Lodge, Arkenfield, Ross-on-Wye HR9 5BB. Tel: 01989 567359.

Homeopathy

The British Homeopathic Association 27a Devonshire Street, London W1N 1RJ. Tel: 0171 935 2163. Will supply a list of medically qualified doctors who are also qualified in homeopathy, and pharmacists stocking homeopathic medicines. SAE required.

The Society of Homeopaths 2 Artizan Road, Northampton NN1 4HU. Tel: 01604 21400.

There are five NHS homeopathic hospitals to which you can be referred to by your doctor:

The Bristol Homeopathic Hospital Cotham Road, Bristol BS6 6JU. Tel: 0117 973 1231.

The Glasgow Homeopathic Hospital 1000 Great Western Road, Glasgow G12 0NR. Tel: 0141 211 1600.

The Liverpool Homeopathic Clinic The Department of Homeopathic Medicine, The Mossley Hill Hospital, Park Road, Liverpool L18. Tel: 0151 250 3000.

The Royal London Homeopathic Hospital Great Ormond Street, London WC1 3HR. Tel: 0171 837 8833.

The Tunbridge Wells Homeopathic Hospital Church Road, Tunbridge Wells, Kent. Tel: 01892 542977.

Hypnotherapy

British Hypnotherapy Association 1 Wythburn Place, London W1H 5WL. Tel: 0171 723 4443. For information send £5.

British Society of Medical and Dental Hypnosis 42 Links Road, Ashtead, Surrey KT21 2HJ. Tel: 01372 273522.

Medical Herbalism

The National Institute of Medical Herbalists 56 Longbrook Street, Exeter EX4 6AH. Tel: 01392 426022. For a list of practitioners send a large SAE (29p stamp).

Osteopathy

The General Council and Register of Osteopaths 56 London Street, Reading RG1 4SQ. Tel: 01734 576585. Will supply a list of registered osteopaths. Please send an SAE.

Reflexology

Association of Reflexologists 27 Old Gloucester Street, London WC1N 3XX. Tel: 0990 673320.

Women's Health

Women's Health Information Centre 52–54 Featherstone Street, London EC1Y 8RT. Tel: 0171 251 6580.

General Health

Action on Pre-Eclampsia (APEC) 31–33 College Road, Harrow, Middlesex HA1 1EJ. Tel: 01923 266778.

Active Birth Movement 25 Bickerton Road, London N19 5JT. Tel: 0171 561 9006.

AIMS 40 Kingswood Avenue, London NW6 6LS. Tel: 0181 960 5585.

Association of Radical Midwives 62 Greetsby Hill, Ormskirk, Lancashire L39 2DT. Tel: 01695 572776.

Cry-sis B.M. Cry-sis, London WC1N 3XX. Helpline: 0171 404 5011. If you would like information please send an SAE.

Foresight (pre-conceptual care) 28 The Paddock, Godalming, Surrey GU7 1XD. Tel: 01483 427839.

The Foundation for the Study of Infant Deaths 14 Halkin Street, London SW1X 7DP. Helpline: 0171 235 1721. Info: 0171 235 0965. Fax: 0171 823 1986.

Galen Homoeopathics Lewell Mill, West Stafford, Dorchester, Dorset DT2 8AN. Tel: 01305 263996.

Gingerbread (single parents) 49 Wellington Street, London WC2E 7BN. Tel: 0171 240 0953.

Independent Midwives Association Nightingale Cottage, Shamblehurst Lane, Botley, Southampton SO32 2BY. Tel: 01703 694429

London Hazards Centre (advice on occupational hazards in pregnancy) Interchange Studios, Dalby Street, London NW5 3NQ. Tel: 0171 267 3387. For free fact sheets, send an SAE (London area only).

MAMA (Meet-a-Mum Association) 14 Willis Road, Croydon CR0 2XX. Tel: 0181 665 0357.

Maternity Alliance 45 Beech Street, London EC2P 2LX. Tel 0171 588 8582.

Miscarriage Association c/o Clayton Hospital, Northgate, Wakefield, West Yorkshire WF1 3JS. Tel: 01924 200799.

National Caesarean Support Network c/o Sheila Tunstall, 2 Hurst Park Drive, Huyton, Liverpool L36 1TF. Tel: 0151 480 1184.

National Childbirth Trust Alexandra House, Oldham Terrace, Acton, London W3 6NH. Tel: 0181 992 8637.

National Child Minding Association 8 Mason's Hill, Bromley, Kent BR2 9EY. Tel: 0181 464 6164.

National Council for One Parent Families 255 Kentish Town Road, London NW5 2LX. Tel: 0171 267 1361.

(P6) TENS
Hire from: **Neen Healthcare (TNS)** Old Pharmacy Yard, Church Street, Dereham, Norfolk NR19 1DJ. Tel: 01362 698966

Parents Anonymous 8 Manor Gardens, London N7 6LA. Tel: 0171 263 8918.

Parents at Work 77 Holloway Road, London N7 8JZ. Helpline: 0171 700 5771.

Pregnancy Advisory Service 11–13 Charlotte Street, London W1P 1HD. Tel: 0171 637 8962.

Relaxation for Living (relaxation techniques) 12 New Street, Chipping Norton, Oxfordshire OX7 5LJ. Tel: 01608 646100.

Stillbirths and Neonatal Deaths Society 28 Portland Place, London W1N 4DE. Tel: 0171 436 5881.

Support After Termination for Abnormality 73 Charlotte Street, London W1P 1LB. 0171 631 0280. Helpline: 0171 631 0285.

Twins and Multiple Birth Association PO Box 30, Little Sutton, South Wirral L66 1TH. Tel: 0151 348 0020.

VBAC Information and Support (vaginal birth after Caesarean) Linda Howes, 8 Wren Way, Farnborough, Hampshire GU14 8SZ. Tel: 01252 543250.

Women's Environmental Network 22 Highbury Grove, London N5 2EA. Tel: 0171 354 8823.

Suppliers of herbs and essential oils by post

G. Baldwin and Co. 173 Walworth Road, London SE17 1RW. Tel: 0171 703 5550.
Neal's Yard Apothecary 15 Neal's Yard, Covent Garden, London WC2H 9DP. Tel: 0171 379 7222. Also supplies homeopathic remedies (reasonably priced).
D. Napier and Sons Ltd (mail order) Forest Bank, Barr, Ayrshire KA26 9TN. Tel: 01465 861625.
Self-Heal Herbs Hayes Corner, South Cheriton, Templecombe, Somerset BA8 0BR. Tel: 01963 370300.
Aqua Oleum (oils) Unit 3, Lower Wharf, Wallbridge, Stroud, Glos. GL5 3JA. Tel: 01453 753555.

Sickness bags

You can buy personal waste bags, as sickness bags are known, from the following supplier. They come in three sizes and lots of either 250 or 500, depending on the size. The codes with which to order them are DRB SO 2498 (small), DRB SO 2499 (medium), and DRB SO 2501 (large). From: 3S Healthcare, Arterial House, 313 Chase Rd, Southgate, London N14 6JH. Tel: 0181 920 6206

Sea-bands

Available by post from Novafon Ltd, 3 Atholl Road, Pitlochry PH16 5BX. Tel: 01796 472735.

FURTHER READING

Stephen Davies and Alan Stewart, *Nutritional Medicine*. Pan Books 1987
C. Lessell, *Biochemic Handbook*. Thorsons 1984
Denise Tiran, *Complementary Therapies for Pregnancy and Birth*. Baillière Tindall 1995
Nicky Wesson, *Alternative Maternity*. Vermilion 1995
Patsy Westcott, *Alternative Health Care for Women*. Thorsons 1987

Acupuncture

Julian Kenyon, *Acupressure Techniques*. Thorsons 1987

Aromatherapy

Allison England, *Aromatherapy for Mother and Baby*. Vermilion 1993
Maggie Tisserand, *Aromatherapy for Women*. Thorsons 1990

Homeopathy

Miranda Castro, *Homeopathy for Mother and Baby*. Macmillan 1992
Drs Sheila and Robin Gibson, *Homeopathy for Everyone*. Penguin 1991

Massage

Clare Maxwell Hudson, *The Complete Book of Massage*. Dorling Kindersley 1988
Stephen Russel and Yehudi Gordon, *Massage for Life*, available by post from 156 Hendon Way, London NW2 0NE at £3.40, including postage and packing

Medical Herbalism

Juliette de Bairacli Levy, *The Illustrated Herbal Handbook*. Faber 1982
David Hoffman, *The New Holistic Herbal*. Element MA USA 1991
Anne McIntyre, *Herbs for Pregnancy and Childbirth*. Sheldon Press 1988
Michael McIntyre, *Herbal Medicine for Everyone*. Penguin 1990
Earl Mindell, *The Herb Bible*. Vermilion 1994
Daniel Reid, *Chinese Herbal Medicine*. Thorsons 1987
Carol Rogers, *A Woman's Guide to Herbal Medicine*. Hamish Hamilton 1995
Susun Weed, *The Wise Woman Herbal for the Childbearing Year*. Ash Tree Publishing, USA 1985, available from Compendium Books, 234 Camden Street, London NW1 8QS

Reflexology

Inge Dougans and Suzanne Ellis, *Art of Reflexology*. Element Books 1992
Kevin and Barbara Kunz, *Complete Guide to Foot Reflexology*. Thorsons 1984

REFERENCES

Anderson AS. 1994. Managing pregnancy sickness and hyperemesis gravidarum. *Professional Care of Mother and Child*, Vol. 4, No. 1. pp. 13–15.

(anon). 1994. Indian herbs used in pregnancy, birth and breastfeeding. *Birth Traditions Survival Bank Newsletter*, Vol. 4, No. 1. pp. 7–9.

Apfel R, Kelly S, Frankel F. 1986. The role of hypnotizability in the pathogenesis and treatment of nausea and vomiting of pregnancy. *Journal of Psychosometric Obstetrics and Gynaecology*, Vol. 5. pp. 179–86.

Arthurs G. 1994. Hypnosis and acupuncture in pregnancy. *British Journal of Midwifery*, Vol. 2, No. 10. pp. 495–98.

Atkinson W. 1882. Treatment of the vomiting of pregnancy. *Obstetric Gazette*, Vol. 5. pp. 596–600.

Atlee H. 1934. Pernicious vomiting of pregnancy. *Journal of Obstetrics and Gynecology*, Vol. 41. pp. 750–59.

Avon. 1992. *Children of the Nineties*. MIDIRS, June, p. 155.

Baram DA. 1995. Hypnosis in reproductive health care: a review and case reports. *Birth*, Vol. 22, No. 1. pp. 37–42.

Bashiri A, Neumann L, Maymon E, Katz M. 1995. Hyperemesis gravidarum: epidemiologic features, complications and outcome. *European Journal of Obstetrics and Gynecology and Reproductive Biology*, Vol. 63. pp. 135–38.

Baylis J, Leeds A, Challacombe D. 1982. Persistent nausea and food aversions in pregnancy. *Clinical Allergy*, Vol. 13. pp. 263–69.

Beal M. 1992. Acupuncture and related treatment modalities. Part II: Applications to Antepartal and Intrapartal Care. *Journal of Nurse Midwifery*, Vol. 37, No. 4.

Belluomini J, Litt RC, Lee KA et al. 1992. Acupressure for nausea and vomiting of pregnancy: a randomised, blinded study. *Obstetrics and Gynecology*, Vol. 80, No. 5. pp. 852–54.

BiSoDol. 1932. Vomiting of pregnancy: a symposium of the current literature. New Haven: BiSoDol Company.

Boericke W. 1927. *Materia Medica*. Philadelphia PA: Boericke and Runyon.

Borison HL. 1989. Area postrema: chemoreceptor circumventricular organ of the medulla oblongata. *Progress in Neurobiology*, Vol. 32. pp. 351–90.

Bourne G. *Pregnancy*. Pan Books.

Brandes JM. 1967. First trimester nausea and vomiting as related to the outcome of pregnancy. *Obstetrics and Gynecology*, Vol. 30. pp. 427–31.

British National Formulary. 1996. London: British Medical Association and Pharmaceutical Press.

Burton J. 1751. *An essay towards a Complete New System of Midwifery, Theoretical and Practical*. Printed for James Hodges, at the Looking-Glass, facing St Magnus' Church, London.

Burton J. 1751. *Essays towards a Complete New System of Midwifery – Theoretical and Practical*.

Coperman 1875. In Schjott-Rivers E. Hyperemesis gravidarum: clinical and biological investigations. *Acta Obstetrics and Gynecology*, Scand, 18 suppl. 1–4, pp. 1–245.

Coppen A and Brist M. 1959. Vomiting of early pregnancy: psychological factors and body build. *Lancet*, Vol. 2. pp. 172–73.

Culpepper N. 1651. *Directory for Midwives*.

Curtis A. 1837. *Obstetrics, Lectures on Midwifery and the Forms of Disease Peculiar to Women and Children*. Columbus, Ohio: Jonathan Philips.

Czeizel AE, Dudas I, Fritz G and others. 1992. The effect of periconceptional multivitamin-mineral supplementation on vertigo, nausea and vomiting in the first trimester of pregnancy. *Archives of Gynecology and Obstetrics*, Vol. 251. pp. 181–85.

Dally A. 1982. *Inventing Motherhood*. London: Burnett Books.

Davies S and Stewart A. 1987. *Nutritional Medicine*, Pan Books.

De Aloysio D, Penacchioni P. 1992. Morning sickness control in early pregnancy by Neigan Point acupressure. *Obstetrics and Gynecology*, Vol. 80, No. 5. pp. 852–54.

Department of Health. 1994. *Folic acid and the prevention of neural tube defects*. Report from Expert advisory Group for the DOH, 1994. available from: Health Publication Unit, Heywood Stores, No. 2 Site, Manchester Road, Heywood, Lancashire OL10 2PZ.

Depue K, Dernstein L, Ross K, Judd I, Henderson D. 1987. Hyperemesis gravidarum in relation to estradiol levels, pregnancy outcome, and other maternal factors: seroepidemiologic study. *American Journal of Obstetrics and Gynecology*, Vol. 156. pp. 1147–51.

Dilorio C. 1985. First trimester nausea in pregnant teenagers: Incidence, characteristics, intervention. *Nurs. Res.* Vol. 34. pp. 372–77.

DuBois P. 1852. *Bulletin d'Académie Médicine*. Vol. 17, No. 557. Paris.

Duncan J and Harding V. 1918. A report on the effect of high carbohydrate feeding on the nausea and vomiting of pregnancy. *Journal of the Canadian Medical Association*, Vol. 8. pp. 1057–69.

Dunlop et al. 1982. Maternal haemoglobin concentration, haematocrit and renal handling of urate in pregnancies ending in the births of small-for-dates infants. *Obstetrics and Gynaecology Survey*, Vol. 37, No. 11. pp. 649–940.

Evans A, Samuels SN, Marshall C, Bertolucci LE. 1993. Suppression of pregnancy-induced nausea and vomiting with sensory afferent stimulation. *Journal of Reproductive Medicine*, Vol. 38, No. 8. pp. 603–606.

Fagan EA and Chadwick VS. 1983. Drug treatment of gastrointestinal disorders in pregnancy. In *Lewis PJ ed. Clinical Pharmacology in obstetrics*. Bristol. Wright PSG 114–37.

Fairweather D. 1965. Hyperemesis gravidarum. MD Thesis, University of St Andrew's.

Fairweather D. 1968. Nausea and vomiting in pregnancy. *American Journal of Obstetrics and Gynecology*, Vol. 102, No. 1. pp. 135–75.

Fairweather D. 1978. Nausea and vomiting during pregnancy. *Obstetrics and Gynecology Annual*, Vol. 7. pp. 91–105.

Fen Cheung N. 1996. Chinese diet therapy in childbirth. *Midwives*, Vol. 109, No. 1301. pp. 146–49.

Fischer-Rasmussen et al. 1990. *European Journal of Obstetrics and Gynaecology and Reproductive Biology*, Vol. 38. pp. 19–24.

Flaws B. 1983. *Path of Pregnancy*. Massachusetts: Paradigm Publications.

Ford JM. 1986. Homeopathy in pregnancy. *Midwives Chronicle and Nursing Notes*, June. pp. 185–87.

Fox D. 1834. *The Signs, Disorders and Management of Pregnancy: the Treatment to be Adopted During and After Confinement; and the Management and Disorders of Children*. London: Henry Mosely.

Freeland-Graves J. et al. 1980. *Journal of the American Dietetic Association*, Vol. 77.

Godfrey K, Robinson S, Barker DJP and others. 1996. *British Medical Journal*, Vol. 312, No. 7028. pp. 410–14.

Goldenberg RL. 1996. Prepregnancy weight and pregnancy outcome. *Journal of the American Medical Association*, Vol. 275, No. 14.

Goldstein L. 1996. Homeopathic remedies for morning sickness. In: Pathos M, Heimlich J. *Homeopathic medicine at home*. The Birthkit. p. 7.

Gross S, Librach C, Cecutti A. 1989. Maternal weight loss associated with *hyperemesis gravidarum*: a predictor of fetal outcome. *American Journal of Obstetrics and Gynecology*, Vol. 160, No. 4. pp. 906–909.

Guillemeau J. 1612. *Childbirth or the Happy Deliverie of Women*. London: Hatfield.

Harries JM, Hughes TF. 1958. Enumeration of some of the 'cravings' of some pregnant women. *British Medical Journal*, July, pp. 39–40.

Harvey W and Sherfey M. 1954. Vomiting in pregnancy: a psychiatric study. *Psychosomatic Medicine*, Vol. 16. pp. 1–9.

Henker F. 1970. Psychotherapy as adjunct in treatment of vomiting during pregnancy. *South Medical Journal*, Vol. 69. pp. 1585–87.

Hook EB. 1978. Dietary cravings and aversions during pregnancy. *American Journal of Clinical Nutrition*, Vol. 31. pp. 1355–62.

Howden C. 1986. Prescribing in pregnancy: treatment of common ailments. *British Medical Journal*, Vol. 293. pp. 1549–50.

Huft PS. 1980. Safety of drug therapy for nausea and vomiting of pregnancy. *J. Fam. Pract*, Vol. 11, pp. 969–70.

Hutton E. 1988. Sickness in pregnancy. *New Generation*, Vol. 7, No. 1, pp. 9–10.

Hyde E. 1989. Acupressure therapy for morning sickness: a controlled clinical trial. *Journal of Nurse-Midwifery*, Vol. 34. pp. 171–78.

Jarnfelt-Samsioe A, Eriksson B, Walderstrom J, Samsioe G. 1985. Some new aspects on emesis gravidarum: relations to clinical data, serum electrolytes, total protein and creatinine. *Gynecologic Obstetric Investigations*, Vol. 19. pp. 174–86.

Jarnfelt-Samsioe A, Eriksson B, Walderstrom J, Samsioe G. 1986. Serum bile acids, gamma-glutamyl transferase and routine liver tests in emetic and non-emetic pregnancies. *Gynecologic Obstetric Investigations*, Vol. 21. pp. 169–76.

Jarnfelt-Samsioe A, Samsioe G, Velinder G. 1983. Nausea and vomiting in pregnancy: a contribution to its epidemiology. *Gynecologic Obstetric Investigations*, Vol. 16. pp. 221–29.

Kallen B. 1987. Hyperemesis during pregnancy and delivery outcome a registry study. *European Journal of Obstetrics and Gynecology and Reproductive Biology*, Vol. 26. pp. 291–302.

Kaltenbach K. 1891. *Ztschr. Geburtsh. v. Gynäk*, Vol. 21. p. 200.

Kaplan B. 1994. Homeopathy: 2 – In pregnancy and for the under-fives. *Professional Care of Mother and Child*, August/September 1994. pp. 185–87.

Kenyon J. 1987. *Acupressure techniques. Self-help guide*. London: Thorsons.

Klebanoff MA, Koslowe PA, Kaslow R, Rhoads GC. 1985. Epidemiology of vomiting in early pregnancy. *Obstetrics and Gynecology*, Vol. 66. pp. 612–16.

Klebanoff MA, Mills JL. 1986. Is vomiting in pregnancy teratogenic? *British Medical Journal*, Vol. 292. p. 724.

Kloss J. 1985. *Back to Eden*. Back to Eden book 1. Loma Linla, California: Back to Eden Books.

Koller O. 1982. The clinical significance of hemodilution during pregnancy. *Obstetrics and Gynaecology Survey*, Vol. 37, No. 11. pp.649–52.

Korte D. 1995. Morning Sickness serves a purpose. *Mothering*, Winter. pp. 20–21.

Kousen M. 1993. Treatment of nausea and vomiting in pregnancy. *American Family Physician*, Vol. 48, No. 7, pp. 1279–83.

Kullander S, Kallen B. 1976. A prospective study of drugs and pregnancy II: anti-emetic drugs. *Acta. Obstet. Gynecol. Scand.*, Vol. 55. pp. 105–11.

Lawless J. 1992. *Encyclopaedia of Essential Oils*. London: Element Books.

Lewis PJ and Chamberlain GVP. 1982. Treatment of everyday complaints in pregnancy. *Prescriber's Journal*, Vol. 22, pp. 77–84.

Lim KB, Hawkins DF. 1989. Management of common disorders during pregnancy. *Postgraduate Update*, Vol. 39, No. 5.

McCammon C. 1951. A study of four hundred seventy five pregnancies in American Indian women. *American Journal of Obstetrics and Gynecology*, Vol. 61. pp. 1159–66.

Meyer MB, Jonas BS, Tonascia JA. 1976. Perinatal events associated with maternal smoking during pregnancy. *American Journal of Epidemiology*, Vol. 103. pp. 464–76.

Miklovich L, van den Berg BJ. 1976. An evaluation of the teratogenicity of certain antinauseant drugs. *American Journal of Obstetrics and Gynecology*, Vol. 129. pp. 244–48.

Minturn L, Weiher A. 1984. The influence of diet on morning sickness: a cross-cultural study. *Medical Anthropology*, Vol. 8. pp. 71–75.

Montgomery W. 1837. *An Exposition of the Signs and Symptoms of Pregnancy, the Period of Human Gestation, and the Signs of Delivery.* London: Sherwood, Gilbert and Piper.

Mowrey DB, Clayson DE. 1982. Motion sickness, ginger and psychophysics. *Lancet*, Vol. 1. pp. 655–57.

National Academy of Sciences. 1989. *Recommended Dietary Allowances (10th edn)*. Washington DC: National Academy Press.

Nelson MM, Forfar JO. 1971. Association between drugs administered in pregnancy and congenital abnormalities of fetus. *British Medical Journal*, Vol. 1. pp. 523–27.

Newman V, Fullerton J, Anderson P. 1993. Clinical advances in the management of severe nausea and vomiting during pregnancy. *Journal of Obstetric, Gynecologic and Neonatal Nursing*, Vol. 22, No. 6. pp. 483–90.

O'Brien B, Naber S. 1995. Nausea and vomiting during pregnancy: effects on the quality of women's lives. *Birth*, Vol. 22, No. 2, pp. 93–100.

O'Brien B, Newton N. 1991. Psyche versus soma: historical evolution of beliefs about nausea and vomiting during pregnancy. *Journal of Psychosometric Obstetrics and Gynaecology*, Vol. 12, pp. 91–120.

O'Brien B, Zhou Q. 1992. Variables related to nausea and vomiting during pregnancy. *Birth*, Vol. 19, No. 3, pp. 138–43.

Pettitti D. 1986. Nausea and pregnancy outcome. *Birth*, Vol. 13. pp. 223–26.

Pickard, B. 1982. *Nausea and vomiting in early pregnancy*. Self-publication, p. 2.

Pickard, B. 1984. *Eating Well for a Healthy Pregnancy*. Sheldon Press.

Pitman V. 1994. *Herbal Medicine*. Shaftesbury, Dorset: Element Books.

Posner LB, McCottry, Posner AC. 1957. Pregnancy cravings and pica. *Obstetrics and Gynecology*, Vol. 9. pp. 270–72.

Priest J. 1990. *Drugs in Pregnancy*. London: Pandora Press.

Reid DP. 1987. *Chinese Herbal Medicine*. London: Thorsons Books. p. 116.

Robertson G. 1946. Nausea and vomiting of pregnancy: a study in psychosomatic and social medicine. *Lancet*, Vol. 2. pp. 366–46.

Ross W (ed). 1988. Aristotle II i Encyclopaedia Britannica. C Chicago: *Encyclopaedia Britannica*. pp. 108–11.

Rumeau-Roquette C, Goujard J, Huel G. 1977. Possible teratogenic effect of phenothiazines on human beings. *Teratology*, Vol. 15. pp. 57–64.

Sahakian V, Rouse D, Siper S, Rose N et al. 1991. Vitamin B6 is effective therapy of nausea and vomiting of pregnancy: a randomized, double-blind, placebo-controlled study. *Obstetrics and Gynecology*, Vol. 78. pp. 33–36.

Semmens J. 1971. Female sexuality and life situations: an etiologic, psycho-socio, sexual profile of weight gain and nausea and vomiting in pregnancy. *Obstetrics and Gynecology*, Vol. 38. pp. 555–63.

Shapiro S, Kauffman DW, Rosenberg L et al. 1978. Meclozine in pregnancy in relation to congenital malformations. *British Medical Journal*, Vol. 1, p. 487.

Sheehan HL. 1939. *Journal of Obstetrics and Gynaecology*. British Empire, Vol. 46, p. 685.

Slone D, Siskind V, Heinonen OP, Monson RR et al. 1977. Ante-natal exposure to the phenothiazines in relation to congenital malformations, perinatal mortality rate, birthweight and intelligence quotient score. *American Journal of Obstetrics and Gynecology*, Vol. 128. pp. 486–88.

Smellie W. 1779. *Treatise on the Theory and Practice of Midwifery, book 2*. London.

Stainton MC, Neff EJA. 1994. The efficacy of seabands for the control of nausea and vomiting in pregnancy. *Health Care for Women International*, Vol. 15, No. 6, pp. 563–75.

Stapleton H. 1995. The use of herbal medicine in pregnancy and labour: part 1 – an overview of current practice. *Complementary Therapies in Nursing and Midwifery*, Vol. 1. pp. 148–53.

Tanner T. 1868. *On the Signs and Diseases of Pregnancy*. London: Henry C Lea.

Taylor DJ. et al. 1976. Haematological changes during normal pregnancy: iron-induced macrocytosis. *British Journal of Obstetrics and Gynaecology*, Vol. 83. pp. 760–67.

Temkin O. 1956. *Soranus' Gynaecology*. Baltimore: Johns Hopkins Press.

Tierra M. 1980. *The Way of Herbs*. London: Orenda/Unity Press.

Tiran D, Mack S. 1995. *Complementary Therapies for Pregnancy and Childbirth*. London: Bailière Tindall.

Titus P, Givens M. 1920. The role of carbohydrates in the treatment of toxaemias of early pregnancy. *Journal of the American Medical Association*, Vol. 14. pp. 777–83.

Tyack AJ. 1991. Vomiting in pregnancy. *Current Obstetrics and Gynecology*, Vol. 1. pp. 93–96.

Van Lier D, Manteuffel B, Dilorio C, and others. 1993. Nausea and fatigue during early pregnancy. *Birth*, Vol. 20, No. 4, pp. 193–97.

Van Stuijvenberg, Schabort I, Labadorious D, Nel J. 1995. The nutritional status and treatment of patients with hyperemesis gravidarum. *American Journal of Obstetrics and Gynecology*, Vol. 172, No. 5. pp. 1585–91.

Vaughan. 1789. *Memoirs of the Medical Society*. Vol. 2, No. 125. London.

Vickers AJ. 1996. Can acupuncture have specific effects on health? A systematic review of acupuncture antiemesis trials. *Journal of the Royal Society of Medicine*, June. pp. 303–11.

Whang R, Whang DD, Ryan MP. 1992. Refractory potassium depletion: a consequence of magnesium deficiency. *Archives of Internal Medicine*, Vol. 152. pp. 40–45.

Whitehead SA, Andrews DLR, Chamberlain GUP. 1992. Characterisation of nausea and vomiting in early pregnancy: a survey of. *Journal of Obstetrics and Gynaecology*, Vol. 12, No. 6, pp. 364–69.

Winkler L. 1985. Drugs in pregnancy: is there an alternative? *Parents*, June, pp. 14–15.

Winn D. 1996. The truth about morning sickness. *She* magazine's *Having a Baby*. Spring/Summer. p. 23.

Wolkind S and Zajicek E. 1978. Psycho-social correlates of nausea and vomiting in pregnancy. *Journal of Psychosomatics*. RCS, Vol. 22. pp. 1–5.

Zhao RJ. 1987. Thirty nine cases of morning sickness treated with acupuncture. *Journal of Traditional Chinese Medicine*, Vol. 7. pp. 25–26.

INDEX